The Pharmacy Technician Series

COMPOUNDING

Series Author
Mike Johnston, CPhT

Contributing Authors
Linda F. McElhiney, PharmD., R. Ph.
Brenda Pavlic, CPhT
Robin Luke, CPhT

The Pharmacy Technician Series
The Pharmacy Technician Series
The Pharmacy Technician Series
The Pharmacy Technician Series
The Pharmacy Technician Series

PEARSON
Prentice Hall

pper Saddle River, New Jersey 07458

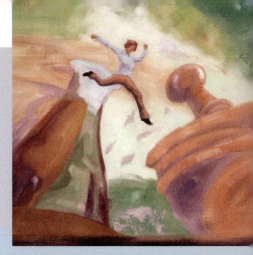

Library of Congress Cataloging-in-Publication Data
The pharmacy technician series. Compounding / [edited by] Mike Johnston.
p. cm.
Includes bibliographical references and index.
ISBN 0-13-114760-9 (alk. paper)
1. Drugs—Dosage forms.— 2. Pharmacy technicians. I. Johnston, Mike, CPhT.
[DNLM: 1. Drug Compounding. 2. Dosage Forms. QV 778 P53572 2006]
RS200.P45 2006
615'.19—dc22 2005045933

National Pharmacy Technician Association

The NPTA logo is a trademark of the National Pharmacy Technician Association

straden-schaden, inc.®

RxPRESS PUBLICATIONS®

The Straden-Schaden and RxPress logos are both trademarks of Straden-Schaden, Inc.

Publisher: Julie Levin Alexander
Assistant to Publisher: Regina Bruno
Acquisitions Editor: Joan Gill
Developmental Editor: Triple SSS Press Media Development, Inc.
Editorial Assistant: Bronwen Glowacki
Director of Marketing: Karen Allman
Marketing Coordinator: Michael Sirinides
Channel Marketing Manager: Rachele Strober
Director of Production and Manufacturing: Bruce Johnson
Managing Production Editor: Patrick Walsh
Production Liaison: Christina Zingone
Production Editor: Rosaria Cassinese/Prepare, Inc.
Manufacturing Manager: Ilene Sanford
Manufacturing Buyer: Pat Brown
Design Director: Cheryl Asherman
Interior Designer: Amy Rosen
Cover Designer: Mary Siener
Cover Illustrator: Edward Sherman
Compositor: Prepare, Inc.
Printer/Binder: Courier/Kendallville
Cover Printer: Phoenix Color Corp.
Photo Acknowledgment: We wish to thank the National Pharmacy Technician Association, Multi Med Media, and Jeremy Van Pelt (photographer).
Chapter 1 opening photo: © Getty Images, Inc., Photodisc
Cover Illustration: © 2006 by Edward Sherman

Notice: The author and the publisher of this volume have taken care to make certain that the doses of drugs and schedules of treatment are correct and compatible with the standards generally accepted at the time of publication. Nevertheless, as new information becomes available, changes in treatment and in the use of drugs become necessary. The reader is advised to carefully consult the instruction and information material included in the package insert of each drug or therapeutic agent before administration. This advise is especially important when using, administering, or recommending new and infrequently used drugs. The author and publisher disclaim all responsibility for any liability, loss, injury, or damage incurred as a consequence, directly or indirectly, of the use and application of any of the contents of this volume. It is the responsibility of the reader to familiarize himself or herself with the policies and procedures set by the federal, state, and local agencies as well as the institution or agency where the reader may be employed. It is the reader's responsibility to stay informed of any new changes or recommendations made by any federal, state, and local agency as well as by his or her employing institution or agency.

Pearson Education Ltd.
Pearson Education Singapore Pte. Ltd.
Pearson Education Canada, Ltd.
Pearson Education—Japan
Pearson Education Australia Pty. Limited
Pearson Education North Asia Ltd.
Pearson Educación de Mexico, S.A. de C.V.
Pearson Education Malaysia Pte. Ltd.

PEARSON Prentice Hall

10 9 8 7 6 5 4 3 2
ISBN 0-13-114760-9

Dedication

In loving memory of Bob Cummings . . . my Papa.

Victor Hugo once wrote, "there is no grandfather who does not adore his grandson." I believe that to be true, just as much as this grandson adored his grandfather.

Our time together on earth was short lived, but the time we spent together has created a lifetime of cherished memories.

Here is to . . . glass bottled cokes . . . Hostess fried pies . . . Del Dixie pickles . . . the yellow parakeet . . . and insight that can come only from a grandfather.

Contents

The Pharmacy Technician Series

The Pharmacy Technician Series

The Pharmacy Technician Series

The Pharmacy Technician Series

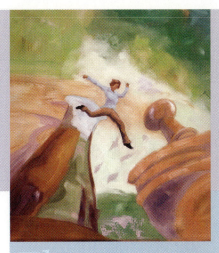

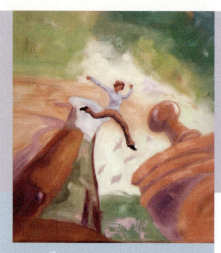

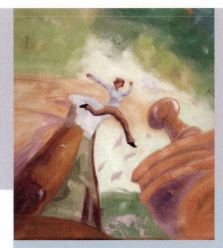

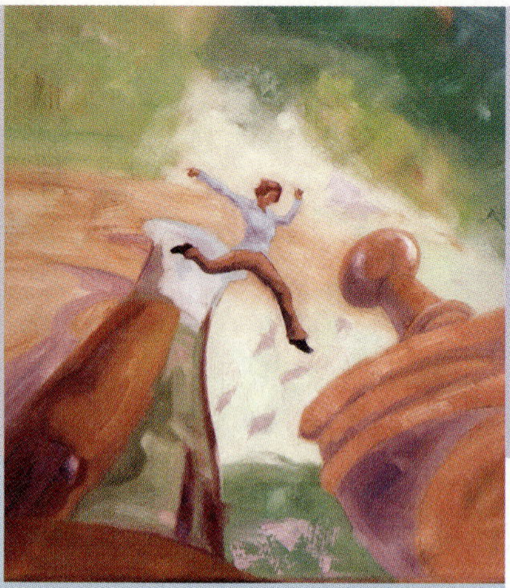

The Pharmacy Technician Series

The Pharmacy Technician Series
The Pharmacy Technician Series
The Pharmacy Technician Series

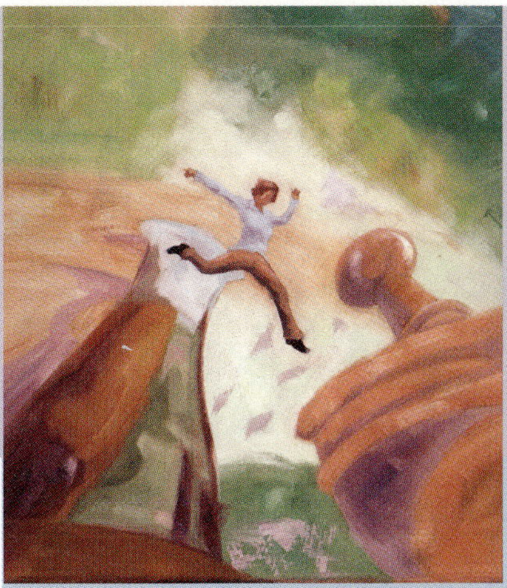

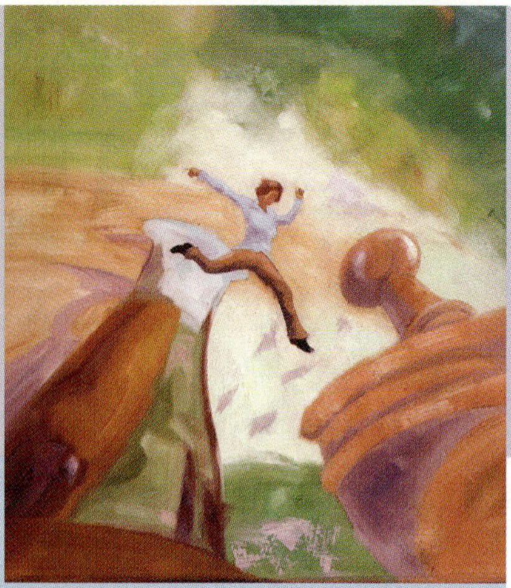

The Pharmacy Technician Series

The Pharmacy Technician Series
The Pharmacy Technician Series
The Pharmacy Technician Series

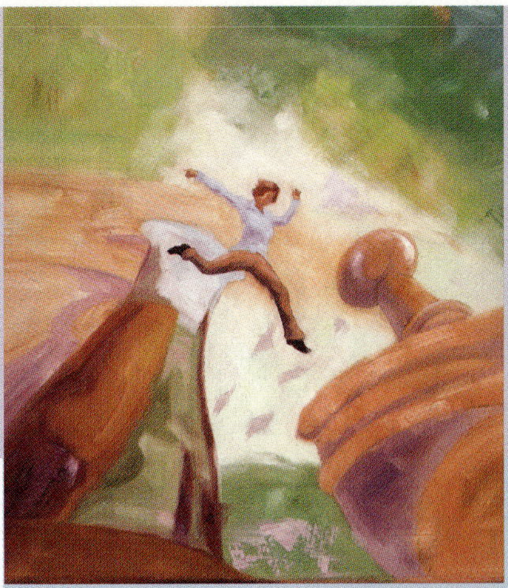

The Pharmacy Technician Series

The Pharmacy Technician Series

The Pharmacy Technician Series

The Pharmacy Technician Series

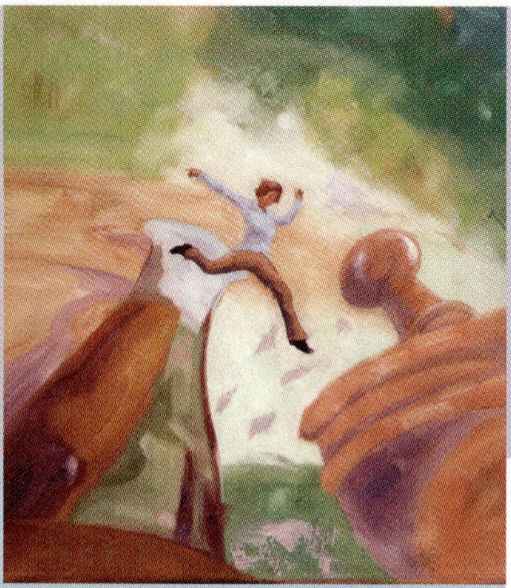

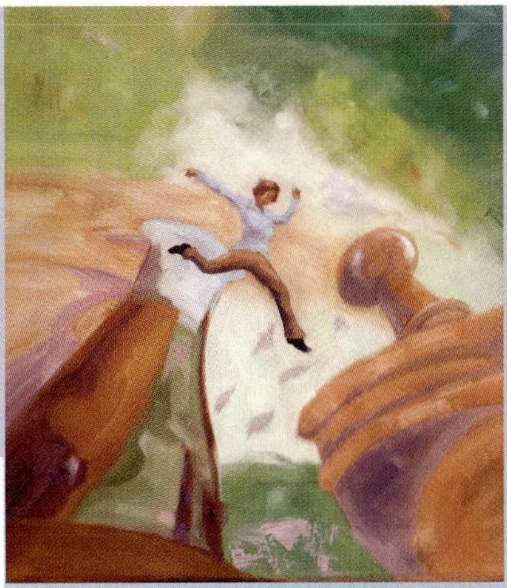

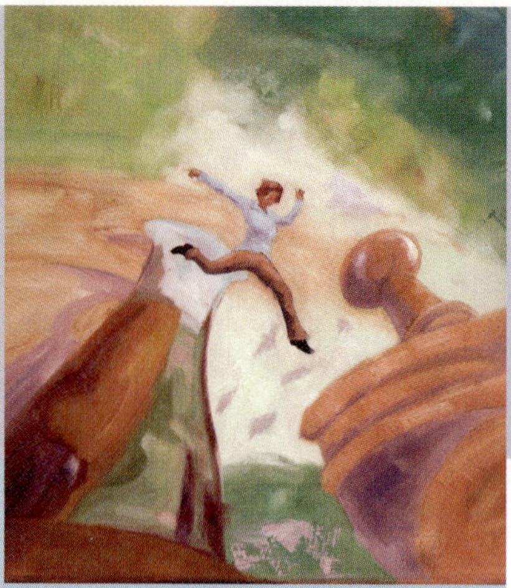

The Pharmacy Technician Series

The Pharmacy Technician Series
The Pharmacy Technician Series
The Pharmacy Technician Series

Preface

Compounding is a core title in Prentice Hall's newest series for pharmacy technician education. *The Pharmacy Technician Series* comprises six books that have been developed and designed together, ensuring greater success for the pharmacy technician student.

About the Book

Pharmaceutical compounding is not only a science, but also an art; while not all pharmacies practice this art, the demand for patient-specific medications is increasing rapidly. This means new career opportunities are developing for pharmacy technicians.

This book is detailed—so detailed, in fact, that it will serve as a dependable reference manual in many pharmacies. The book, however, has also been designed to guide the student through with ease, as each theory builds upon those presented in earlier chapters.

The core features of this book include the following:

- Chapter introductions and summaries provide the student with a clearer understanding and rationale of the content being covered.
- Logical, step-by-step instructions with full-color photos direct the student in compounding virtually every type of dosage form.
- Workplace Wisdoms provide quick, highlighted tips and comments that replicate the advice of a seasoned compounding professional.
- Practice Formulas covering each of the major dosage forms addressed allow students or trainees to practice and master each compounding technique.
- Chapter Reviews provide a mechanism for both the student and instructor to assess concept comprehension.
- Practical Examples provided throughout the text serve as a comprehensive overview; these appear as case studies common to actual practice settings to better prepare the pharmacy technician student.

About the Series

While there are a variety of textbooks and training manuals available for the pharmacy technician, none meets the true educational needs of the industry. Accordingly, in this volume we set out to develop the most comprehensive, accurate, and current texts ever published for pharmacy technicians. One method we used to achieve this goal was involving pharmacy technician educators and trainers from across the country in every phase of the project. Each title in this series has been developed, written, and reviewed by practicing pharmacy technician educators and practicing pharmacy professionals—a winning approach.

About the Authors

Linda F. McElhiney, PharmD., R.Ph.

Linda is the compounding pharmacist for Clarian Health Partners in Indianapolis, Indiana. She oversees the entire compounding and repackaging operations for the three hospitals and the outpatient clinics within the Clarian system.

Linda was instrumental in designing a new compounding laboratory, computerizing compounding operations, and establishing a PharmD rotation in compounding for Purdue and Butler Universities. As a result of her dedication, Purdue appointed Linda as an affiliate assistant professor of clinical pharmacy, and Butler appointed her as an affiliate associate professor for the College of Pharmacy.

Brenda Pavlic, CPhT

Brenda is a certified pharmacy technician with over 20 years of experience. In 2001, she became co-owner of SaveWay Compounding Pharmacy in Delaware. Prior to this, Brenda worked in independent and chain retail pharmacies, where she served as lead technician and pharmacy department manager.

In 2002, Brenda specialized in compounding by completing a comprehensive course offered by the National Pharmacy Technician Association (NPTA) and the Professional Compounding Centers of America (PCCA). A few of the many duties that she performs in her current setting include calculations, determining the best dosage form, compounding, training, researching stability, determining solubility, and sourcing chemicals needed to prepare compounds.

Robin Luke, CPhT

Robin is a founding member of NPTA's Executive Advisory Board—the elected body of leaders for the National Pharmacy Technician Association. She has over 10 years of experience in institutional pharmacy, sterile product preparation, compounding, bulk-manufacturing and management, with a specialized knowledge of herbals and homeopathic treatments.

Robin has developed a variety of continuing education programs, with a strong emphasis on reducing medication errors; she also speaks at meetings and conferences across the United States.

with

Mike Johnston, CPhT

Mike is known internationally as a respected author and speaker in the field of pharmacy. He published his first book, *Rx for Success—A Career Enhancement Guide for Pharmacy Technicians*, in 2002.

In 1999, Mike founded NPTA in Houston, Texas, and led the association in growth from 3 members to over 20,000 in less than two years. Today, as executive director of the National Pharmacy Technician Association and publisher of *Today's Technician* magazine, he spends the majority of his time meeting with and speaking to employers, manufacturers, association leaders, and elected officials on issues related to pharmacy technicians.

About NPTA

NPTA, the National Pharmacy Technician Association, is the world's largest professional organization established specifically for pharmacy technicians. The association is dedicated to advancing the value of pharmacy technicians and the vital roles they play in pharmaceutical care. In a society of countless associations, we believe it takes much more than a mission statement to meet the professional needs and provide the required leadership for the pharmacy technician profession—it takes action and results.

The organization is composed of pharmacy technicians practicing in a variety of settings, such as retail, independent, hospital, mail-order, home care, long-term care, nuclear, military, correctional facility, formal education, training, management, sales, and many more. NPTA is a reflection of this diverse profession and provides unparalleled support and resources to members.

NPTA is the foundation of the pharmacy technician profession; we have an unprecedented past, a strong present, and a promising future. We are dedicated to improving our profession while remaining focused on our members.

For more information on NPTA:
Call 888-247-8700
Visit www.pharmacytechnician.org

Acknowledgments

This book, which is part of a six-title series, has been both an exhilarating and an exhausting project. To say that this series is the result of a collaborative team effort would be a gross understatement.

Special thanks to SaveWay Compounding Pharmacy (Bear, Delaware), PCCA (Professional Compounding Centers of America, Houston, Texas), and Clarian Health System (Indianapolis, Indiana) for your assistance with this text. Nearly every photograph presented throughout this book was shot on location at your facilites. We are grateful for the assistance, patience, and collaboration of your entire staff.

We would also like to thank Jeremy Van Pelt (Photographer) and Multi Med Media (Production Management).

Mark — thank you for believing in my initial vision and concept for this series, which was anything but traditional. I will always remember the day we spent in New York City talking about cover concepts and the like at coffee shops and art galleries. More importantly, I am honored to have gotten to know you, Alex and now little Sophie—and I consider each of you friends.

Joan — you are truly gifted at what you do. I am amazed at your ability to join this project at the point you did and to guide each daunting task to a smooth and successful accomplishment. I feel that your leadership has created a better final product.

Julie — thank you for taking risks (plural) on this project, boldly departing from standard policies and procedures. In the end, your support and belief allowed a truly innovative product to be published.

Robin — your commitment to this project—to exceeding all expectations, to developing the best training series for pharmacy technicians available—has been amazing. You are a wonderful, gifted individual; but most importantly, I am thankful to call you a friend.

Andrew and Jenny — thank you for supporting this project, each in your own unique way; thank you for supporting me and the entire organization. This project tested each of us—our character and our will—and I am honored to know you both.

Most importantly, I wish to thank my family. The past several years have been difficult and trying, but the strength, love, and support that you have given me have always pulled me through. ***Thank you***.

Reviewers

The reviewers of The Pharmacy Technician Series have provided many excellent suggestions and ideas for improving these texts. The quality of the reviews has been outstanding, and the reviews have been a major aid in the preparation of the manuscript. The assistance provided by these experts is deeply appreciated.

Lisa C. Barnes, B. Pharm, M.B.A.
ACPE Program Administrator,
Adjunct Assistant Professor
of Pharmacy Practice
University of Montana School of Pharmacy and Allied Health Sciences
Missoula, Montana

Kimberly Brown, CPh.T.
Associate Director and Instructor
of Pharmacy Technology
Walters State Community College
Morristown, Tennessee

Ralph P. Casas, Pharm. D., Ph.D.
Associate Professor of Pharmacology
Cerritos Community College
Norwalk, California

Kristie Fitzgerald, B.S., Pharm
Clinical Pharmacist, Department
of Neonatology; Instructor
Salt Lake Community College
Salt Lake City, Utah

Madeline Jensen-Grauel, B.S., Ed., M.Sc.
Director, Pharmacy Technician Training Program
The University of Texas Medical Branch at Galveston
Galveston, Texas

Robert D. Kwiatkowski, B.S., M.A.
Adjunct Instructor
PIMA Medical Institute
Colorado Springs, Colorado

Herminio Maldonado, Jr., M.S., B.S.
Pharmacy Technician Instructor
PIMA Medical Institute
Colorado Springs, Colorado

Bradley Moore, MSN
Director of Health Science
Remington Administrative Services, Inc.
Little Rock, Arkansas

Hieu Nguyen, B.S., CPh.T.
Pharmacy Technician Program Director
Western Career College
Sacramento, California

CHAPTER 1

Introduction to Compounding

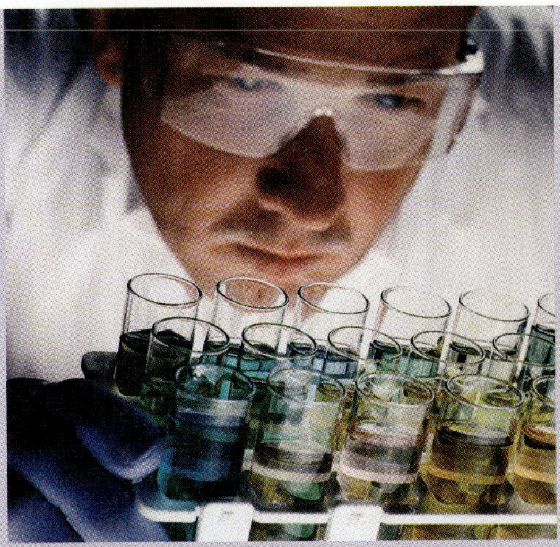

Learning Objectives

After completing this chapter, you should be able to:

- Explain the reasons why compounding is a vital part of pharmacy practice.
- List different types of compounding formulations.
- Identify specific considerations for patient care and compounding.
- Describe various patient types that commonly use compounds.
- Discuss the role of pharmacy technicians in compounding.

INTRODUCTION

There is a steadily increasing need for **compounding** in pharmacy practice today. Pharmaceutical compounding is the practice of extemporaneously preparing medications to meet the unique need of an individual patient on the basis of the specific order of a prescriber.

Every pharmacy setting at some point will compound a prescription. It may be as simple as combining two topical ingredients to create a preparation with a dual function in an approach to healing. In other cases, compounding will be an extensive and complex procedure of combining more than one active ingredient with several **excipients** to produce a desired product.

Why Compound?

compounding
to produce or mix by combining two or more parts.

excipients
any more or less inert substance added to a prescription in order to confer a suitable consistency or form to the drug; a vehicle.

There are many reasons why the art and science of compounding are being practiced more and more in today's pharmacy practice setting. Some drugs have been discontinued by their manufacturer. Although the medications are no longer commercially available, there are some patients who still require them. Other drugs have been pulled from the market by the Food and Drug Administration. These drugs may have other "off-label" uses and therefore may be compounded at the pharmacy level. A few medications whose active ingredients are no longer suitable for human use are effectively used to treat certain diseases in animals.

Types of Compounds

Pharmacy is the only profession that allows the extemporaneous compounding of chemicals for therapeutic care. There are several common dosage forms that can be prepared by a compounding pharmacy. Capsules, liquids, transdermal gels, creams, ointments, suppositories, troches, quick dissolving tablets, and chewables are just a few of the unique dosage forms that can be offered. Each of these dosage forms requires precise instructions for preparing. The form chosen will depend on how the prescription is ordered, the physical properties of the drug being ordered, the best route of administration according to the individual patient, and availability of the active ingredient.

Capsules and liquids are oral dosage forms that can be formulated to contain the exact strength needed for the patient's required dose. If a patient requires several medications to be compounded, it may be advantageous to combine these therapies into one compounded prescription, reducing the actual number of doses being administered and offering the patient or care giver a more convenient dosing regimen. However, research must be done to ensure compatibility of not only the active ingredients but also any excipients used in the final formulation. A compounding pharmacy can also formulate capsules to contain a lowered dose of the required drug, avoiding the cutting of a tablet into halves or quarters, which may result in a sub-therapeutic or super-therapeutic dose. This also ensures that maintenance medications are exact on a daily basis with regard to the patient's weight and disease state.

Patient Considerations

lactose intolerant
unable to digest dairy-based foods.

For complete patient care, many factors must be taken into consideration. The most important of these factors is the patient. It is imperative to get to know the patient so that the most appropriate dosage form can be offered to ensure compliance and patient safety. A complete patient profile must be collected from the patient or the patient's care giver. This should include all of the patient's allergies and sensitivities, not just those that are drug related. A **lactose intolerant** patient should have his medications prepared with an excipient other than lactose, such as avicel, which will not cause a negative reaction for the patient. Possibly no filler at all is necessary so that the avoidance of a problem is guaranteed. The same is true for the patient who may have sensitivities or allergies to certain preservatives. These things must be determined before any compound can be considered.

PEDIATRICS

The pediatric patient needing a medication that is currently available only in an adult formulation may require this particular medication to be compounded into a palatable liquid and offered in a dose that is appropriate to the young patient. Another option may be to compound the prescription into a topical cream or transdermal gel, offering a less invasive approach to administering the medication. This is an especially good choice for the very young, the mentally or physically challenged, the elderly, or the animal patient to ensure compliance with a needed therapy regimen. Patients with a gastrotube or naso-gastrotube require all of their medications to be in liquid form. Many of these medications are not commercially available as a liquid; therefore, they must be compounded.

Children with autism, depending on the degree of their disease, can be especially difficult to medicate. Trying to medicate with an oral product can often result in extreme trauma, confusion, and fear. Many parents of these children are unable to medicate them successfully or consistently. Daily vitamins, sleep aids, and other medications can be compounded in a topical form that is administered in a soothing fashion or in a pleasant tasting oral form that the patient will readily take. Current protocols for treating the autistic child call for medications without preservatives or certain other ingredients. Although the total amount dispensed may have to be reduced due to stability considerations, these meds can be formulated by leaving out the agent(s).

TERMINALLY ILL PATIENTS

Hospice patients or the terminally ill are other groups that can benefit greatly from utilizing a compounding pharmacy. Many of these patients are unable to swallow oral medications. Again, preparing their medications in topical form will improve compliance as well as reduce the stress involved in administration for both the patient and the person caring for him. Another possibility would be compounding multiple medications into one dosage form, reducing the number of doses to be given.

Cancer patients sometimes develop sores in their mouth as a result of their medications. A compounding pharmacy can prepare a soothing lozenge or lollipop that will bathe the oral cavity with an anesthetic such as lidocaine, bringing temporary relief from the pain associated with the sores. Topical forms of pain medications can be helpful in reducing stomach upset as well as avoiding metabolism by the liver that can lead to hepatic damage.

HOME HEALTH CARE

Home health care is a field that routinely taps into the resources offered by pharmacy compounding. The hospice patient can benefit greatly from compounded prescriptions. His therapies can possibly be combined into one, making dosing easier for both the patient and the care giver. Using topical or transdermal preparations offers the patient a more convenient way to administer the medications needed to treat the symptoms associated with his disease state.

TPNs

Total Parenteral Nutrition
intravenous feeding that provides patients with all essential nutrients when they are unable to feed themselves.

Total Parenteral Nutrition programs and the preparation of intravenous admixtures are areas of medicine that have always relied on compounding. Often, a compounding pharmacy will prepare batches of TPNs for multiple patient use within a facility. IV admixtures are generally made on an as-needed basis. At times, batches may be made in response to a protocol designed for more than one patient suffering from the same disease.

NUCLEAR MEDICINE

volatile
evaporates readily.

Nuclear pharmacy is a specialty area for compounding in pharmacy practice. It consists of compounding and dispensing radioactive materials. Because of the **volatile** and unstable nature of these chemicals, it is often necessary for the chemicals to be compounded just hours prior to use. Most radioactive pharmaceutical doses are delivered to the end user in unit dose form. Special safeguards are used in the nuclear pharmacy. The most common form of protection for the preparer from the hazards of working with these compounds is lead protection. The compounds are usually prepared behind lead glass by using leaded glass syringes as well as lead containers to hold the radioactive materials. Although the potential for risk of contamination is high, these risks can easily be avoided by practicing safe handling techniques. Only a well-trained, supervised pharmacy technician will work in the field of nuclear pharmacy.

VETERINARY MEDICINE

Veterinary compounding offers solutions to veterinarians and pet owners alike. Many animals are nearly impossible to dose orally. This creates overwhelming stress to both the owner and the afflicted animal. This added stress can potentially exacerbate the animal's medical condition. Unique dosage forms can be compounded to make giving medication to the animal less difficult. This not only reduces the anxiety involved but also promotes better compliance. Weight is usually the determining factor when prescribing medications for animals. Since there is such a broad range in size among animals, a compounding pharmacy can formulate a prescription that is dose specific to the individual animal.

Formulations currently available only in capsule or tablet form can be compounded into a flavored liquid such as beef, chicken, tuna, or liver, which the animal will more readily take orally. These liquids, flavored in the animal's favorite flavor, may also be mixed with a small amount of food. A flavored oral dosage form that may be compounded is the soft gelatin and food-based chewable. The medicated chewable may be offered as a treat or mixed with a small portion of the animal's favorite food. Another option for veterinary compounding is the rectal suppository. This is especially successful for administering a benzodiazepine during a seizure.

Extremely bitter drugs can be compounded into a transdermal gel which is applied to a hairless area on the animal, such as the pinae of a cat's ear or in the groin area of a dog. If a transdermal gel is the preferred choice of the prescriber or the owner, but the particle size of the drug is greater than the existing hairless area will allow for absorption, then another area, usually the back of the neck, can be shaved to receive the gel.

Role of Pharmacy Technicians in Compounding

In the past, pharmacists were the only ones highly trained in pharmaceutical compounding. Today, pharmacy technicians have the opportunity to learn this art and put it into practice. A willing and competent technician can develop the compounding skills necessary to play an integral role in providing optimum health care to the patient with unique medical needs. The compounding technician can educate himself in pharmaceutical compounding by attending one of many professional training sessions offered.

WORKPLACE WISDOM

The art of compounding is a learned skill, valued by many employers. As with those who possess specialized training and skills in other industries, compounding pharmacy technicians are able to find unique employment opportunities and generally earn incomes higher than the national average for pharmacy technicians.

SUMMARY

Compounding is an established and growing need in contemporary pharmacy practice; it is both an art and a science. A competent and properly trained technician can perform many of the functions involved in preparing a compounded prescription under the supervision and guidance of the pharmacist he is working with.

CHAPTER TERMS

compounding
to produce or mix by combining two or more parts.

excipients
any more or less inert substance added to a prescription in order to confer a suitable consistency or form to the drug; a vehicle.

lactose intolerant
unable to digest dairy-based foods.

Total Parenteral Nutrition
intravenous feeding that provides patients with all essential nutrients when they are unable to feed themselves.

volatile
evaporates readily.

CHAPTER 1

CHAPTER REVIEW QUESTIONS

1. Which profession allows the extemporaneous compounding of chemicals for therapeutic care?
   a. physician
   b. pharmacy
   c. nursing
   d. respiratory therapist

2. Patients with a gastrotube or naso-gastrotube require all of their medications to be in what form?
   a. capsules
   b. patch
   c. liquid
   d. paste

3. Nuclear medicine deals with what type of products?
   a. radioactive
   b. hazardous
   c. neoplastic
   d. electromagnetic

4. A lactose intolerant patient should have his medications prepared with an excipient other than lactose, such as
   a. lidocaine
   b. preservative
   c. avicel
   d. benzodiazepine

5. Which of the following is a dosage form suitable for compounding?
   a. troche
   b. capsule
   c. transdermal gel
   d. all of the above

6. True or false: A patient's sensitivity to sugar, due to diabetes, should be considered when formulating a compound.
   a. true
   b. false

7. True or false: After the FDA has pulled a drug from the market, pharmacies are permitted to compound it for "off-label" uses.
   a. true
   b. false

8. Name four flavors used in compounding that could appeal to animals.

9. List two reasons why compounding is considered a vital part of pharmacy practice.

10. **Critical Thinking** What impact does compounding have in pharmacy? Describe how compounding can improve medication compliance.

Resources and References

1. Allen, Loyd V. Jr., Ph.D. *The Art, Science, and Technology of Pharmaceutical Compounding*. Washington, DC: American Pharmaceutical Association, 1998.
2. Published by IJPC, *International Journal of Pharmaceutical Compounding*. Edmond, OK.
3. Allen, Loyd V. Jr., Ph.D. *Secundum Artem: Pharmacy Compounding Equipment*, Vol. 4, Issue 3. Minneapolis, MN: Paddock Laboratories.
4. Purdue University School of Pharmacy, Division of Nuclear Pharmacy. *What Is Nuclear Pharmacy?* West Lafayette, IN, 2003.

CHAPTER 2

Compounding Practices and Considerations

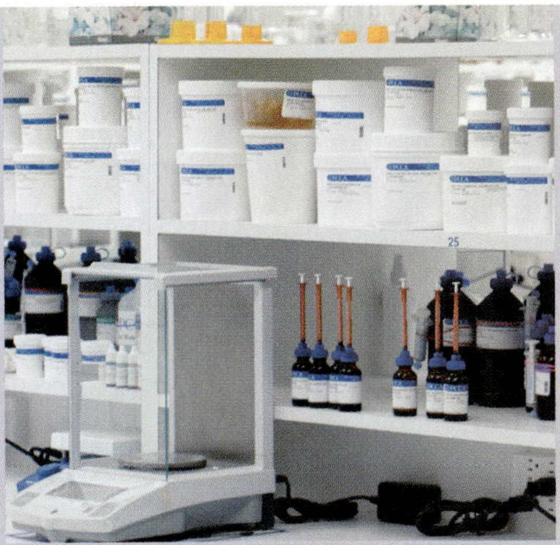

Learning Objectives

After completing this chapter, you should be able to:

- List the factors that must be considered when deciding to compound.
- List the reference books that every compounding pharmacy should have.
- Define and describe solubility, stability, and shelf life.
- Explain general compounding practices.
- List general guidelines to follow when determining expiration dates.

INTRODUCTION

The profession of pharmacy is as ancient as humankind on earth. It has been associated throughout history with magic, theology, alchemy, crimes, strange occurrences, dogmas, and science. The apothecary is one of the oldest trades or professions listed in the Bible. The compounding procedures developed by the Greek pharmacist-physician, Claudius Galen, are still used today in compounding pharmacies. Currently and throughout history, the compounding pharmacist is the only professional trained to prepare products for the treatment of disease and for cosmetic purposes.

Until the 20th century, all medications were compounded. In the early 1800s, the United States Pharmacopeia (USP) was established to promote standardization of compounded medications. Some pharmacies started applying these standards and began, on a small but increasing scale, to manufacture drug products to meet the growing drug needs of their communities. Eventually, with the Industrial Revolution, these compounding laboratories evolved into pharmaceutical companies that research and manufacture today's drug products.

By the early 1970s, approximately one percent or less of all prescriptions were compounded. Compounding was not very important because the pharmaceutical industry was providing most high quality drug products in a variety of different dosage forms. In the 1980s and 1990s, the number of compounded prescriptions began to increase due to the emergence of home healthcare, hospice care, pain management, and total parenteral nutrition that requires preparations to be compounded to meet the specific needs of each patient. Many pharmaceutical manufacturers decreased the number of available dosage forms as cost-saving measures for the companies. Most drugs also do not have indications for pediatric patients and are not commercially available in liquid dosage forms for pediatric use.

Compounding has become a very important part of today's pharmacy setting. More and more prescribers are relying on compounding pharmacies and the unique solutions they offer patients with specific needs. Pharmaceutical compounding can be as simple as combining a liquid with a manufactured drug powder to create a suspension, or it can be as complex as preparing a prescription, specifically ordered by a prescriber, which requires many components and labored steps to produce the final product. Compounding differs from traditional pharmacy in that it involves a relationship between the patient, the prescriber, and the pharmacist.

The Art and Science of Compounding

Compounding is often described as being an art form. As with any creative endeavor, when practicing the art of compounding one must pay close attention to detail. The preparer of a compound should be able to interpret a **formulation** and carry out its instructions without error, have a complete understanding of the task, and know what to expect as an end result. It is imperative that the technician be exact with all calculations and measurements. A good compounding technician is one who is careful and concise with every action he performs.

formulation
a recipe or prescription that lists the components and quantities of a product.

DETERMINING WHETHER OR NOT TO COMPOUND

It must first be determined whether a particular prescription can in fact be compounded. There are many factors to be considered in making this determination. Several questions one might ask when considering the possibility of compounding a certain drug include the following:

1. What is the solubility of the active ingredient? Is it soluble? If so, is it soluble in water? in oil? in alcohol?
   Should the drug be suspended? If so, which suspending agent should be used? Is it necessary for a **solvent**, such as glycerin, to be used to wet the drug before suspending?

solvent
capable of dissolving another substance.

2. What is the **stability** of this chemical?
   a. Is it stable in an aqueous solution?
   b. Is it stable in a fixed-oil?
   c. What role does pH play in the stability of the final product?
   d. Do certain excipients affect the chemical adversely with regard to stability?
   e. How do sweeteners and/or flavors affect stability or pH?
   f. What are the storage requirements of the final product?

stability
the state of being stable.

3. Is the active ingredient available for extemporaneous compounding?
   a. Is the active ingredient available in a raw powder form?
   b. Must a commercially prepared product be considered?
   c. If the chemical is only available in a commercial product, can it be manipulated and still retain stability?
   d. Which is more cost-effective for the patient, using the raw chemical powder form of a drug or using a manufactured product?
   e. Which of the two preceding options makes a better product with regard to flavor or consistency?

4. What dosage forms are possible for this particular chemical?

Information Resources

Compounding technicians must have access to the information needed to answer these questions and others concerning the physical properties of the chemicals they are working with. Sources include reference books, journals, articles, and Internet sites. Every pharmacy that compounds prescriptions should have reference materials pertinent to pharmaceutical compounding. The following is a list of books that every compounding pharmacy should have:

- *Remington's Pharmaceutical Sciences.* Mack Publishing Co.
- *The Merck Manual.* Merck Research Laboratories.
- *The Merck Veterinary Manual.* Merck & Co., Inc.
- *Trissel's Stability of Compounded Formulations.* American Pharmaceutical Association.
- *United States Pharmacopeia.* U.S. Pharmacopeial Convention, Inc.
- *Drug Facts and Comparisons.* J.B. Lippincott Co.
- *Veterinary Drug Handbook.* Pharma Vet Publishing.

Compounding Considerations

Every prescription that presents itself as a potential compound requires that at least a minimum amount of information be gathered. As mentioned earlier, the patient's medical profile must be taken into account. It must then be determined whether a particular drug or chemical can in fact be compounded into a quality, efficacious product. Next, research must be done to determine possible sources of the needed drug, stability, cost effectiveness of use, and the best possible choice for the patient. Proper excipients must be chosen with regard to how they may interact either with the patient or with the active ingredient. Flavoring options are determined on the basis of possible **pH** interference or how they may affect stability of the final product.

pH
the symbol relating the hydrogen ion concentration or activity of a solution to that of a given standard solution.

SOLUBILITY

Before any formulation is prepared, research must be done on the drug that is ordered. The solubility of a chemical must be determined. Some chemicals may be suspended in a suspending agent, whereas others must be suspended in fixed oil. Still others must be wet with glycerin before being suspended into a liquid.

STABILITY

Stability is another factor that must be looked at. Even though a drug may be soluble in water, it might not be stable in an aqueous solution. Some chemicals are only stable in a fixed-oil environment. Another consideration with regard to stability is the pH of the final product. Some drugs are stable only at a certain pH level. Therefore, either a basic or an acidic solution may need to be added to adjust the final pH to ensure that it is within the proper limits. Flavoring choices can be affected by the pH as well; therefore, it is important to know the pH of potential flavoring agents being considered.

SHELF LIFE AND STORAGE

shelf life
how long a product is stable until decomposition.

auxiliary labels
supplemental labels that contain important information.

Shelf life and storage requirements for the final product must be taken into consideration when determining the final quantity or volume of the compound that is to be made. Some of the storage requirements that must be communicated to the patient include whether the prescription is to be kept under refrigeration, at room temperature, or protected from light. It is equally important for the consumer that **auxiliary labels** be used that contain instructions that may not be included on the prescription label. These instructions may include directions to shake well before use, use externally, avoid sun exposure, or avoid certain foods or drugs.

Calculations and Formulas

Compounded prescriptions require a number of calculations, a formula or recipe, equipment and supplies, and an area suitable for computing the task.

CALCULATIONS

Most compounded prescriptions require a number of calculations as part of the process for filling and dispensing a prescription. This particular area of compounding has the greatest potential for error. Although most pharmacy math is relatively simplistic, something as minor as a misplaced decimal can have devastating results, including death. The importance of the pharmacy technician's being properly trained and educated in pharmacy calculations is critical to the compounding procedure. Only an individual with a working knowledge and full understanding of pharmacy mathematics should attempt to perform this crucial element of prescription compounding. Even those who are knowledgeable and trained in this area need to double-check themselves or have their calculations confirmed by someone else.

FORMULAS

A formula or recipe for each compounded prescription must be prepared by a pharmacist. From this formula, a worksheet is produced. This may be done either through a computer program or written out thoroughly in legible handwriting. If a computer-based program is used, it is necessary to check the formulation for errors. One should not assume that the information contained in the formula is absolutely correct. As with any computer program, there is potential for error. Like the mortar and pestle, the worksheet is a tool. It should be used as a checkpoint to confirm that calculations were done correctly, total weight or volume is correct, the proper excipient is listed, or the correct unit of measure is expressed. When writing a formula by hand, it is critical to be neat and complete. Every step should be written out so that it is absolutely clear how the compound is to be made. Nothing should be left to be assumed. No abbreviations should be used when listing ingredients. Every quantity should be followed by the appropriate unit of measure. Ditto marks are not acceptable when the previous unit of measure or the same figure for the amount needed is carried forth to the next ingredient. Any amount listed as less than a whole number should be expressed with a lead zero. For example, .1 gm should be written as 0.1 gm.

EQUIPMENT AND SUPPLIES

After the necessary calculations are completed and the desired quantity of ingredients is determined, suitable equipment and supplies should be gathered and delivered to the compounding area. It is important for the compounding technician to know what equipment is available. It is equally important for him to know which tools are most suitable for producing a quality product. Choosing the proper equipment depends on the individual compound to be made. Some of the determining factors for selecting the proper tools include final quantity or volume, steps involved, dosage form, and particle size of the chemical used. It is as important to select the proper size tool as it is to select the proper tool. For example, if the final quantity to be dispensed is 240 ml, then a 2 oz. mortar and pestle would not be of appropriate size to prepare the prescription. The compounding technician should be familiar with available tools and their functions.

FACILITIES AND WORK SPACE

Before a compounded prescription can be prepared, an area suitable for completing the task must be established. This area should be separate from all other work flow. The workspace should be large enough to accommodate the equipment needed, the person preparing the compound, and the necessary ingredients used in making the compound. It should be clear of all debris, clutter, and any other unnecessary items. All tools used in making a compounded prescription should be inspected for cleanliness just before use. This includes but is not limited to balances, spatulas, weigh boats, mortar and pestle, graduates, and beakers. The counter top or surface area should be wiped down with isopropyl 70 percent alcohol or other suitable cleaning solution just before use and again when the compound is complete. This is an important step in the compounding procedure as it guards against cross-contamination as well as ensures that the compound is free of particles that may promote such things as microbial growth in the compound.

General Compounding Practices

Active ingredients and all excipients used in the compound should be collected and placed to the right of the scale. As each ingredient is weighed, the stock bottle should then be moved to the left of the scale. This simple procedure will help to avoid an error, especially in the event that the individual preparing the compound is interrupted. As each ingredient is weighed, the technician should check the label on the chemical and compare it with the formula worksheet. A checkmark should be placed on the formula worksheet, indicating that the correct ingredient was used and that the amount needed was confirmed. The checkmark on the formula worksheet is also an indication that the drug was actually weighed. The weights of active ingredients should be checked by a pharmacist while they are still on the scale. Depending on individual state law, these weights may be checked by another technician.

WORKPLACE WISDOM

It is imperative for avoiding medication errors that good habits are established early and practiced regularly.

Mixing the active ingredient with the excipient(s) should be performed by using the principle of geometric dilution. That is, start with the ingredient of the smallest amount and double the portion by adding the additional ingredients in order of quantity. Each addition should result in a doubled amount until all the ingredients are mixed in. This process ensures even distribution of the active ingredient throughout the final product. Regardless of the type of compound being made, this method should be practiced most of the time.

EXPIRATION DATES

Many times, a formula will give the expiration date along with any special storage requirements. If the expiration date is not given, there are several sources that can be used to determine the recommended beyond-use date. These sources include *Trissel's Stability of Compounded Formulations*, *International Journal of Pharmaceutical Compounding*, the manufacturer's literature, and chemical companies from which the ingredients are purchased.

For the most part, compounded products are made in small quantities, recommended storage is for cool or cold temperatures, and a conservative expiration date is given. If no valid supporting information on stability is available, there are general guidelines that should be followed.

- Compounded liquids in a fixed oil should be stored at room temperature with an expiration date of six months.
- Non-aqueous liquids and solid formulations made from USP grade chemicals should have an expiration date of no later than six months. If the source of drug is a manufactured product, then the beyond-use date should be 25 percent of the product's remaining expiration date or six months, whichever is earlier.
- Aqueous solutions should have an expiration date of 14 days when stored at a cold temperature.
- All other preparations should have an expiration date of 30 days or the intended duration of therapy, whichever is earlier.

PATIENT COUNSELING

When dispensing the compounded prescription to the patient or care giver, it is necessary to discuss with them any important instructions regarding the prescription. For example, if a suspension is made, they need to be instructed not only to shake the bottle well before use, but also to inspect the bottom of the bottle for any sediment. They should also be shown how to dispense a required dose. Storage recommendations should be reviewed. Markings indicating correct dose on oral or topical syringes should be pointed out. This is the final step in compounding a prescription and must be done by a licensed pharmacist.

SUMMARY

The guidelines contained in this chapter are basic and general in nature. The principles discussed may be applied to most compounding situations, but certainly not to all. The purpose of this chapter is to familiarize the technician with some of the compounding basics. All compounding procedures should first be approved by a pharmacist.

CHAPTER TERMS

auxiliary labels
supplemental labels that contain important information.

formulation
a recipe or prescription that lists the components and quantities of a product.

pH
the symbol relating the hydrogen ion concentration or activity of a solution to that of a given standard solution.

shelf life
how long a product is stable until decomposition.

solvent
capable of dissolving another substance.

stability
the state of being stable.

CHAPTER 2

CHAPTER REVIEW QUESTIONS

1. A good compounding technician is one who is __________ and __________ with every action he or she performs.
   a. attractive, smart
   b. older, wiser
   c. careful, concise
   d. none of the above

2. To prevent errors while documenting quantities, what is the rule when it comes to decimals?
   a. Never use a fraction.
   b. Be sure to have the product in stock.
   c. Always use the numeral 0 before any fraction.
   d. Only use whole numbers.

3. The length of time a product is stable until decomposition is called
   a. shelf life
   b. solubility
   c. stability
   d. none of the above

4. Prior to compounding, and once completed, the work surface should be wiped down with
   a. water
   b. cleaning solution
   c. isopropyl 70 percent alcohol
   d. both b and c

5. The process of mixing ingredients by starting with the smallest amount and continuing to double the portion by adding and mixing in the additional ingredients is known as
   a. double mix
   b. geometric dilution
   c. levigation
   d. integration

6. True or false: The level of pH indicates the hydrogen ion concentration or activity of a solution and is crucial in determining stability of a compound.
   a. true
   b. false

7. True or false: Compounded liquids in a fixed oil should be stored at room temperature with an expiration date of one year.
   a. true
   b. false

8. List four resource books that could aid a compounding technician, and briefly describe the usefulness of each.

9. Name five factors to consider when compounding a formulation.

10. **Critical Thinking** Patient counseling is an important aspect of pharmacy service with all prescriptions, but why, in particular, is it so important pertaining to compounded medications?

Resources and References

1. Allen, Loyd V. Jr., Ph.D. *The Art, Science, and Technology of Pharmaceutical Compounding*. Washington, DC: American Pharmaceutical Association, 1998.
2. IJPC, *International Journal of Pharmaceutical Compounding*. Houston, TX.
3. Allen, Loyd V. Jr., Ph.D. *Secundum Artem*. Minneapolis, MN: Paddock Laboratories.
4. Remington, Joseph P. *Remington's Pharmaceutical Sciences*. Easton, PA: Mack Publishing Co., 1985.

CHAPTER 3

Facilities, Equipment, and Supplies

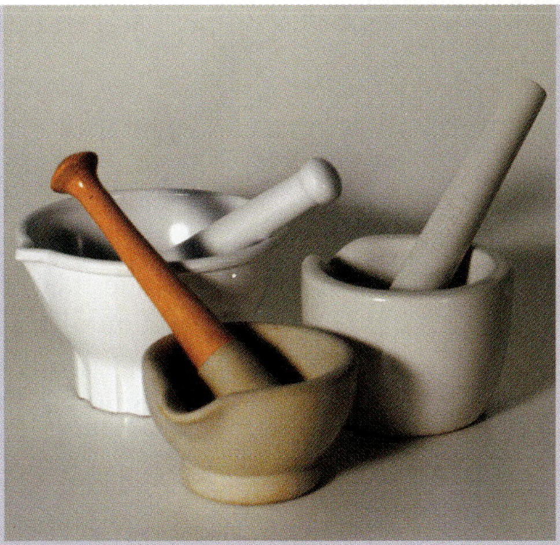

Learning Objectives

After completing this chapter, you should be able to:

- Describe what a compounding facility looks like.
- Identify the equipment contained within a compounding pharmacy.
- List the supplies necessary to extemporaneously compound prescription medication.
- Outline important factors with regard to setting up a facility.
- Specify procedures for maintaining the facility.

INTRODUCTION

The practice of extemporaneous compounding prescription medications has evolved in recent years. With this evolution, the "tools of the trade" have likewise improved. There is still a heavy reliance on the mortar and pestle and other traditionally used pharmaceutical equipment to perform many necessary tasks involved in compounding; but new and more technological advances in equipment and methods have made daily life in the compounding arena easier, more efficient, and quicker and in many situations perhaps lowered the percentages of error associated with compounding. Some of the positive results achieved from using these modern advances are improved patient care, better patient compliance, assurance of exact dosages being administered to the patient, finished products that are of utmost pharmaceutical elegance, more efficacious products offered to prescribers for their patients, easier solutions for problem solving, and increased profit margins.

Facilities

The compounding facility, or laboratory, should be designed in such a way that work processes flow easily and the highest quality products are produced. Of course, space is the major factor when either designing an entire compounding-only facility or simply establishing a compounding area within an existing setting. Regardless of the size and space, certain guidelines should be followed when deciding where and how prescriptions will be compounded (Figure 3-1).

The compounding area should be separate from all other work flow in order for the preparer to be comfortable and away from distractions. It should be kept clean and free of clutter at all times. The area should be well lit and have a controlled temperature as well as proper ventilation. Equipment and supplies frequently used for compounding should be easily accessible. The countertops, floors, walls, ceilings, cabinets, and other matter used to construct the compounding area should be made of materials that will not retain dust, odors, or stains resulting from the compounding process. All surfaces should be smooth, level, and free of any cracks or crevices. Likewise, the surfaces of the **work station** and the cabinets or shelving should be made from products that can be cleaned with minimal effort and cleaning supplies. There shouldn't be any overhangs, hanging light fixtures, exposed pipes, or other such things that can collect dust and dirt possibly contaminating the products that are compounded in the area.

work station
the area defined inside a clean room where the compounding takes place.

CLEANING

All surfaces should be cleaned immediately prior to performing compounding procedures and again at the completion of the task. Likewise, all equipment should be thoroughly examined for cleanliness before use and washed

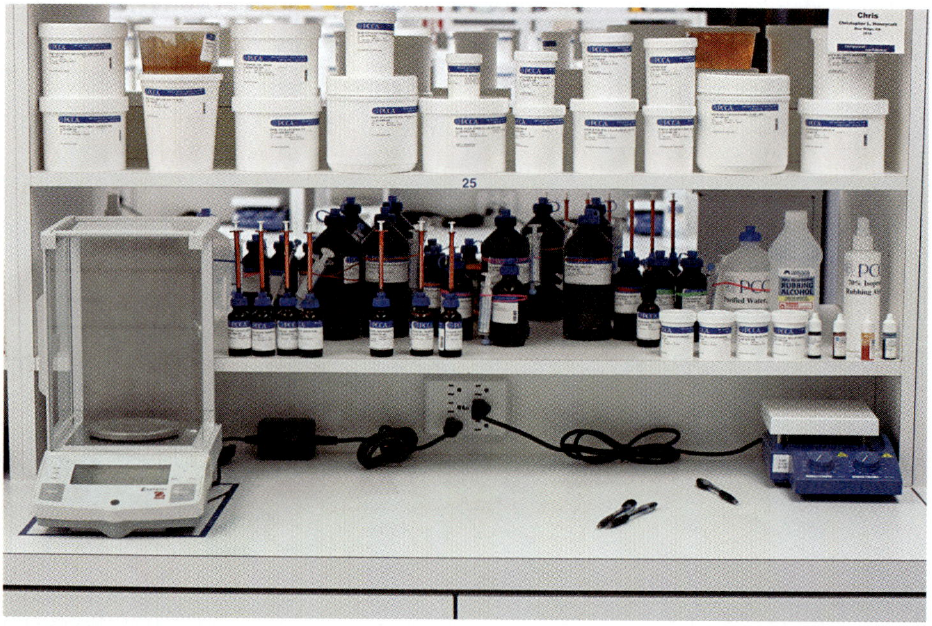

Figure 3-1
Compounding area or room

immediately after use to avoid **cross-contamination** between ingredients and finished products. This includes, but is not limited to, the work surface area and the scale or balance. This process is absolutely critical when working with agents that are caustic or dangerous in nature. The entire compounding area, including floors, walls, and surface areas, should be cleaned thoroughly either daily or weekly. This should be done either at the start of the work day or at the end and never while compounding processes are being performed. It is important to move equipment if possible and clean under and behind, as drug residue may collect there. It is recommended to keep a standard operating procedure (**SOP**) log of each cleaning. If a facility only compounds prescriptions occasionally, pharmacy personnel should perform these tasks prior to any compounding activity.

cross-contamination
when bacteria or particulates migrate to an undesired space and have the potential to cause harm.

SOP
Standard Operating Procedure, a documentation of the operation of a process.

In the selection of cleaning supplies, care must be taken to choose those which will not react with medicinal agents or excipients or contaminate them in any way. This is not quite so critical if cleaning is done at the end of the day, as the solutions will have ample time to dry or evaporate overnight. One appropriate cleaning solution is isopropyl 70 percent alcohol. If sticky residue must be removed, soap and water may be used and then the area wiped down with the alcohol.

An adequate sink with proper drainage and hot and cold running water should be nearby. Cleaning products, sponges, bottle brushes of various sizes, a drainage rack, air driers, and disposable paper towels should be near the washing area. For the larger facility, a dishwasher can prove indispensable, as it will not only thoroughly clean the compounding equipment but may also sterilize it with hot water and heated drying.

DISPOSAL

Trash containers should be kept a distance away from the compounding procedures. All refuse should be disposed of safely and properly. For example, dangerous substances, including disposable gloves, masks, and gowns, should be placed in a zipper bag before disposal. Hazardous waste should not be disposed of in regular trash receptacles, but should be properly bagged and picked up by a company that specializes in hazardous material removal. All trash should be removed from the compounding facility daily. Trash containers should be cleaned on the inside and outside regularly even if they are lined with plastic trash bags.

STORAGE—EQUIPMENT

Items that are commonly used in most compounding procedures, such as mortars and pestles of each type, spatulas, powder scrapers, weigh boats and papers, sieves, beakers, powder funnels, and measuring devices like syringes should be suitably stored in an area that is accessible to each station. Likewise, auxiliary label dispensers, tape dispensers, and prescription bags should be set up for communal use. If possible, these items may be duplicated in more than one place, perhaps in two corner cabinets, where the compounding is performed between the two. These storage compartments should be located out of the way of traffic so multiple preparers won't be interrupting one another during compounding functions. Mortars and pestles, beakers, graduates, and such should be kept in cabinets with doors or turned upside down to prevent dust, dirt, or powder residue from settling inside. Spatulas, powder scrapers, powder or liquid funnels, connectors, adapters, and the like should also be in covered storage such as drawers. The same is true for molds, capsule machines and their plates, and a capsule loader and its plates. If this type of storage condition is not possible, then each piece of equipment should be wiped down with isopropyl alcohol just prior to use and allowed to dry completely before use.

STORAGE—INGREDIENTS

It is also advisable to store the most commonly used drug chemicals and excipients alphabetically in an area that is convenient. Shelving directly above the compounding area would serve this purpose well. Less frequently used ingredients may be stored on shelves or in cabinets in a nearby area. Another section should be established for compounded prescriptions that are made in bulk in the anticipation of repeated use or for refills. These prepared items may be kept with the active ingredients from which they are made or possibly in a drawer cabinet with each drawer labeled with its contents.

All ingredients used in compounding should be stored alphabetically and separated by class. Active powder ingredients should be in one section; powder excipients in another; active liquids in another; and liquid excipients such as diluting agents, wetting agents, solvents, and suspending vehicles in another. A separate section for sterile products (such as injectable products, needles, and syringes) and filters should be in close proximity to where sterile compounding is performed.

Work Stations

If designing a compounding-only facility, it is wise to set up individual stations for the different types of compounded prescriptions. Space limitations, along with a count of the most common types of prescriptions compounded, will determine how many stations are necessary in the facility. There are a few items that should be kept at every station. These include a calculator, weigh boats or papers, spatulas, paper, vinyl or rubber gloves, masks, goggles, and a spray bottle filled with **isopropyl 70 percent alcohol** for cleaning the areas and the tools used in compounding. In addition to these items, a scale or balance used to measure the active ingredients, excipients, or necessary bases should be accessible to each station. If there is a limited number of weighing devices, one may be strategically placed between two stations so it can be shared (Figure 3-2).

isopropyl 70 percent alcohol
an acceptable substance used to wipe down areas to help keep them as clean as possible.

VETERINARY WORK STATION

If chewable veterinary medications are made, they should be compounded in a separate area containing the equipment and supplies used to prepare them. In addition to the items listed above, this area might include mortars and

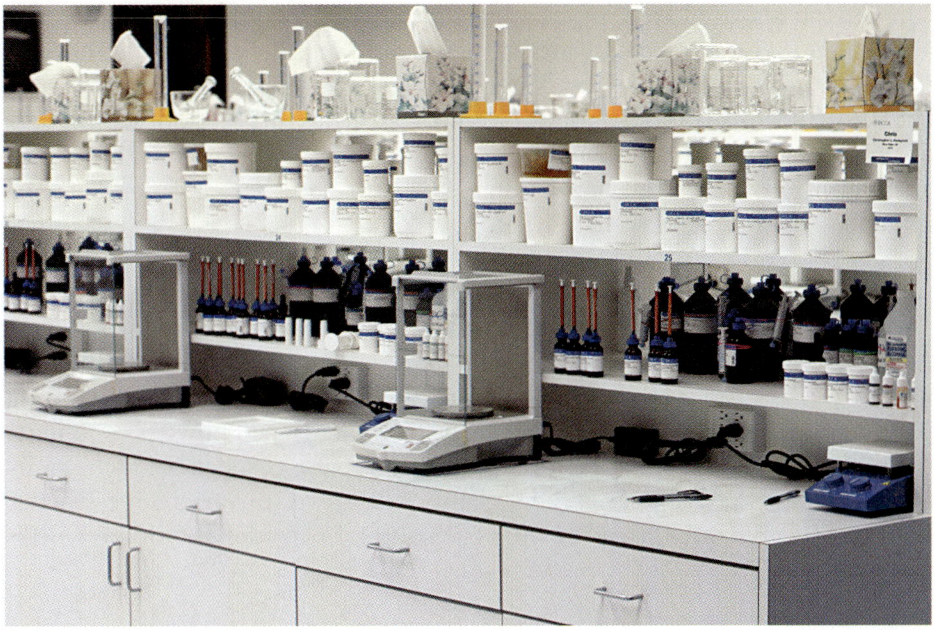

Figure 3-2 Shared equipment at two workstations

pestles, molds specifically manufactured for this purpose, metal and plastic spatulas, Pyrex measuring cups, beakers, and a microwave oven. Other items that should be stored nearby are frequently used medicinal agents, food bases, non-stick cooking spray, a water bottle used to dispense distilled water for polishing the chews, flavoring agents, unit-dose packaging, and a roller used to apply unit-dose labels. This area should have close access to a refrigerator with freezer, as the chews are generally cooled before being removed from the mold.

CREAMS AND OINTMENTS WORK STATION

An area for compounding creams and ointments may have an ointment tile built right into the work surface. If not, an ointment tile should be stored within easy reach, perhaps in a cabinet below. Spatulas, mortars and pestles, commonly used excipients, and active ingredients should all be conveniently placed within reach of the preparer. If an electric mortar and pestle such as an unguator is used, it should be positioned on the counter nearby. This area should also contain ointment jars, tubes, a tube crimper or sealer, bottles, topical syringes, zipper bags, and any other type of container used for the dispensing of creams, ointments, lotions, or transdermal gels. These containers, although usually stored with the lids on, may collect dust or powder residue on the outside and should be cleaned with a disposable paper towel dampened with isopropyl 70 percent alcohol prior to filling.

LIQUIDS WORK STATION

A station designed for the compounding of liquid medications might include a powder funnel, mortars and pestles, a homogenizer, glass stir rods, a magnetic stir plate/hot plate, a liquid blender, beakers, and graduates.

WORKPLACE WISDOM

Organization makes life easier, but in regard to compounding medications it is essential. The more organized and well kept your equipment, ingredients, and work space are, the safer your practice will become. Organization in compounding can aid in preventing medication errors.

distilled water
the most common diluent used in compounding.

WORKPLACE WISDOM

Tap water should never be used in the preparation of a compound. Instead, you must use either distilled water, USP graded water, or SWFI (sterile water for injection).

The excipients used in compounding liquids that should be stored in the area might include distilled water and suspending, diluting, sweetening, and flavoring agents. A device for delivering exact amounts of **distilled water**, such as a Reconstitube®, should be mounted near this station. Containers used for dispensing liquid medications like glass or plastic amber bottles, adaptacaps (if used), and oral syringes dispensed for patient use should be included in this area as well.

CAPSULES WORK STATION

A capsule filling station should include items such as a capsule machine and the various sized plates used with it; a capsule loader and its corresponding plates; empty gelatin capsules in all sizes; frequently used powder excipients such as avicel, dextrose, or lactose; powder scrapers; powder blenders; mortars and pestles of each variety; desiccants; and sieves in various mesh sizes. Vials in multiple sizes used for the dispensing of capsules should be within easy reach.

MOLDS WORK STATION

Molded dosage forms such as suppositories, troches, lozenges, and sticks should be prepared in an area equipped with the necessary molds, a magnetic stir plate/hot plate, beakers, tongs, a thermometer, mortars and pestles, glass stirring rods, hot pads, and a water bottle filled with distilled water. Bases, excipients, and medicinal agents that are used often should be easily accessible to the preparer working in this station. Packaging, such as foil wraps, plastic wraps, lollipop sticks, unit dose packaging, a roller to seal unit-dose labels, cardboard sleeves, and zipper bags in various sizes, should also be kept nearby.

Equipment and Supplies

As noted earlier, the equipment available for the extemporaneous compounding of prescription medication has improved and evolved as the need for such equipment has presented itself. Although these newer tools may have an advantage over traditionally used equipment, there is still a definite need for the time-honored tools of the past. A quality producing compounding laboratory will contain a variety of equipment both new and old. The tools needed and utilized in a specific setting will depend upon the number of prescriptions compounded and the types of most frequently compounded medications performed in the particular setting. Careful study of these factors will determine whether it is advantageous for a compounding pharmacy to invest in certain equipment.

The following is an extensive list of available compounding equipment. Newer and less familiar tools will be defined by their purpose (See Figures 3-3 through 3-66).

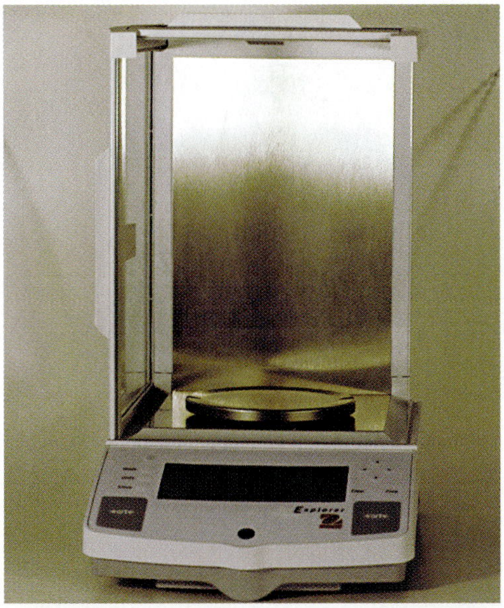

Figure 3-3 Electronic balances are available in various degrees of sensitivity ranging from 1 mg. on up

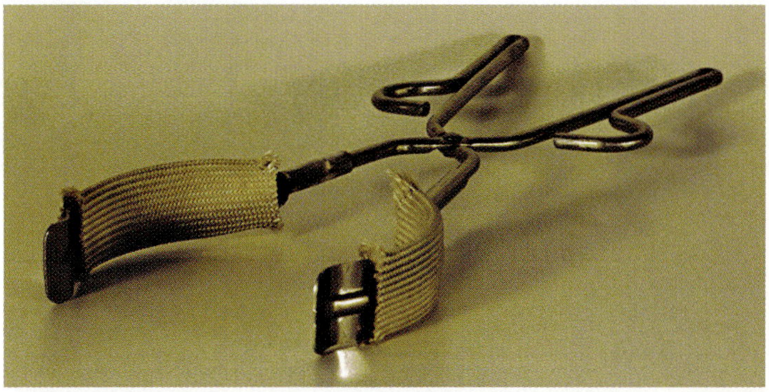

Figure 3-4 Beaker tongs

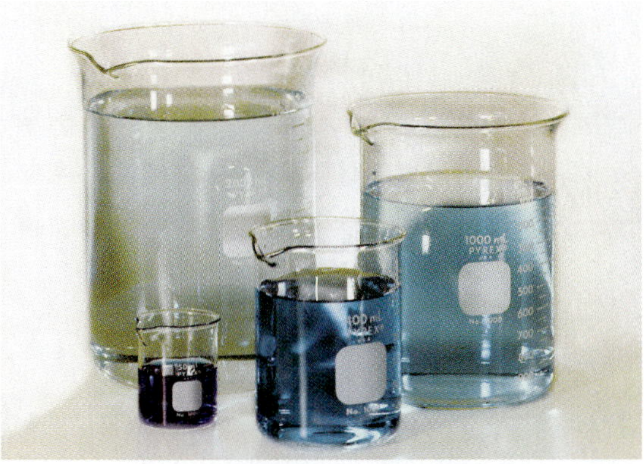

Figure 3-5 Beakers come in various sizes 50, 100, 150, 250, 400, 600, 1000 ml and are made of various materials glass, plastic, stainless steel

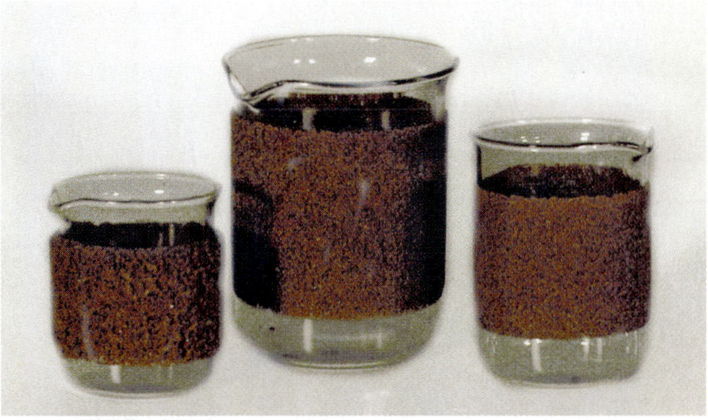

Figure 3-6 Beakers are coated with cork to protect the handler

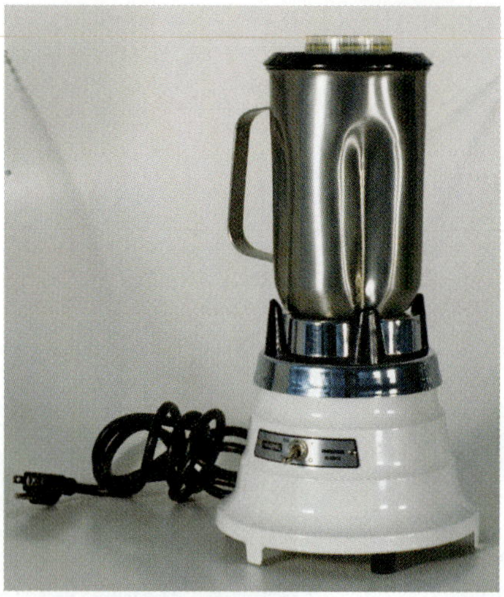

Figure 3-7 Blender used to liquefy, mix, or puree

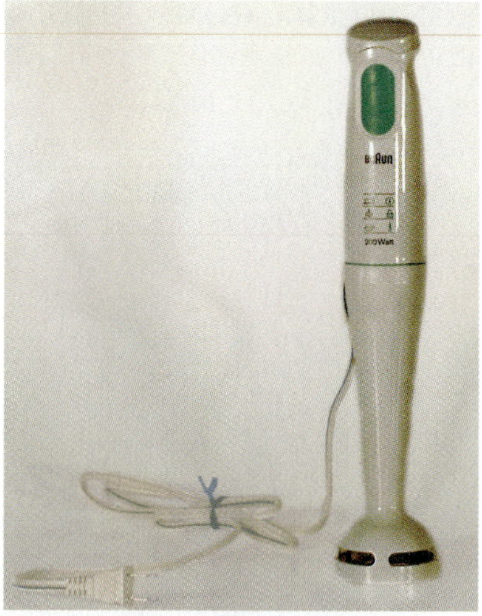

Figure 3-8 Handheld blender for mixing liquids

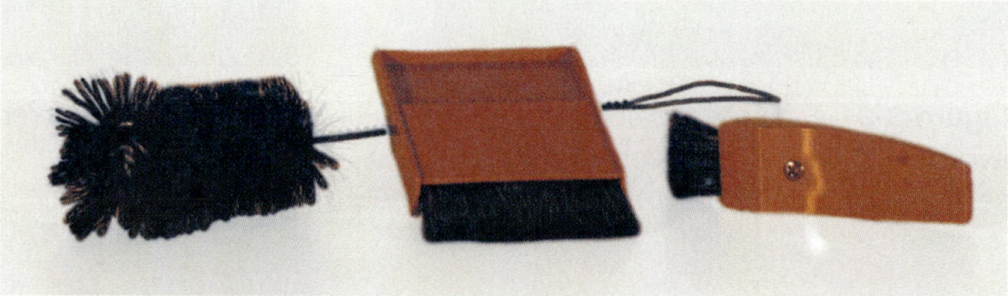

Figure 3-9 Brushes are used for cleaning. Available in many different diameters and lengths

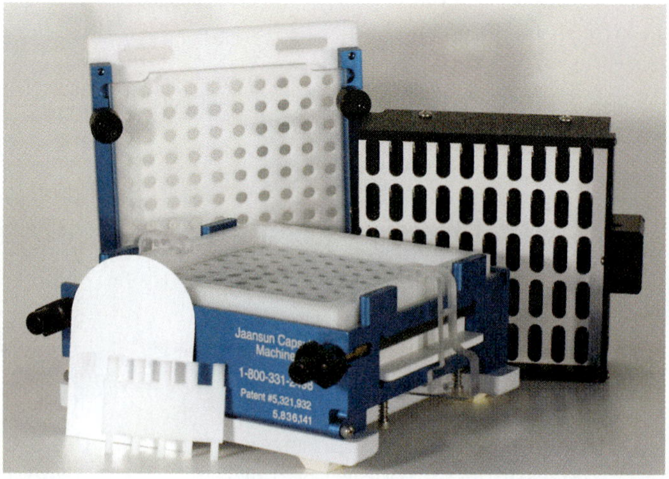

Figure 3-10 Capsule-filling equipment are machines that fill 100 to 300 capsules at a time. Loaders are also available to fill the machine with the empty capsules. Both of these devices have different plate sizes for the various capsule sizes

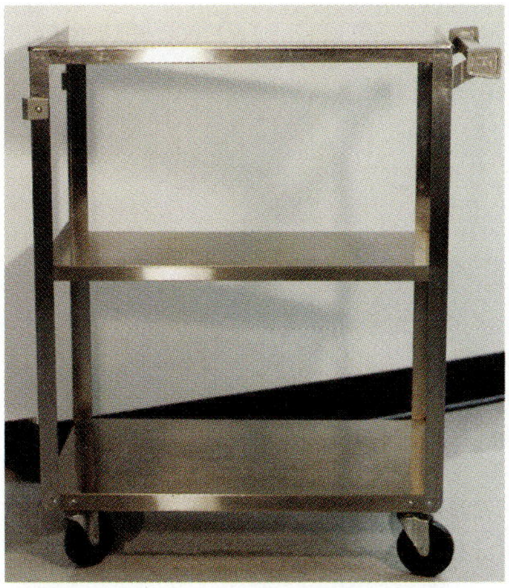

Figure 3-11 Carts come in wood, plastic, or metal

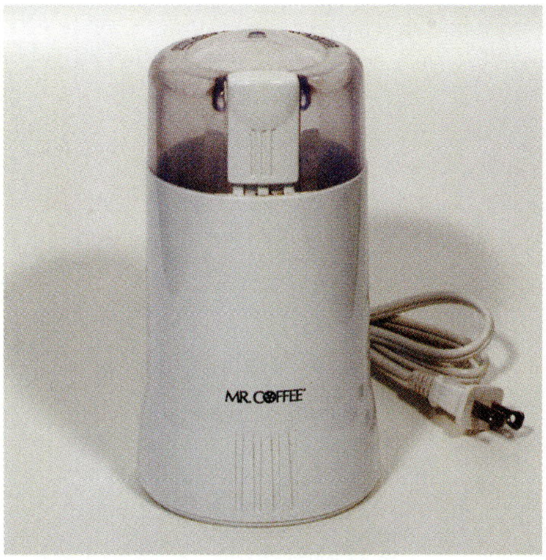

Figure 3-12 Coffee grinder

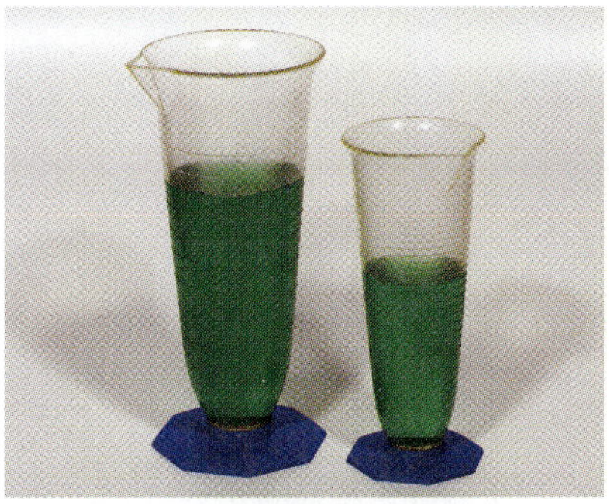

Figure 3-13 Cylinders are graduated 5 ml to 200 ml and can be glass, or plastic

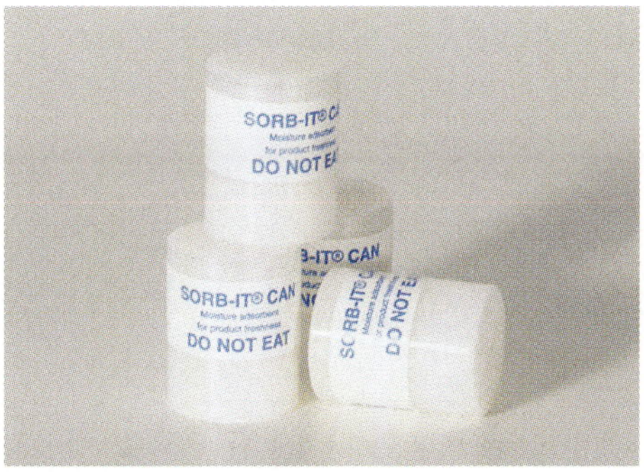

Figure 3-14 Desiccants

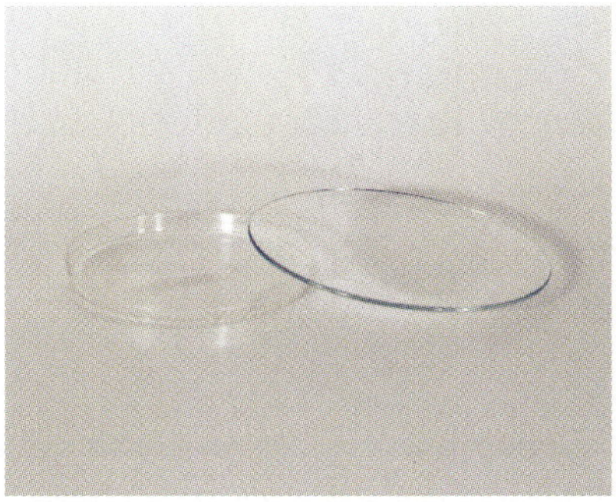

Figure 3-15 Dishes can be evaporating or porcelain and with or without handles

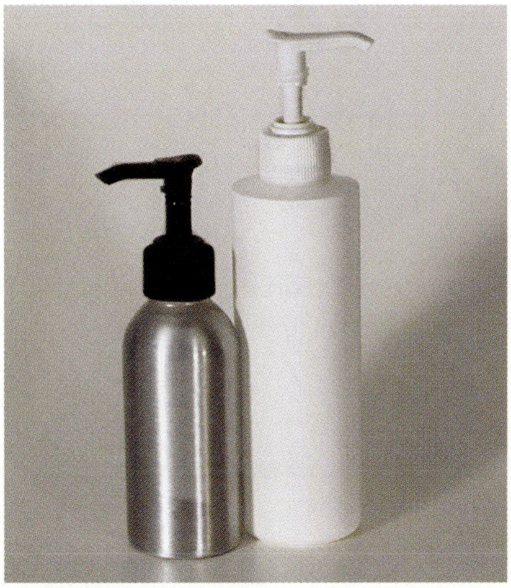

Figure 3-16 Dispensing pumps

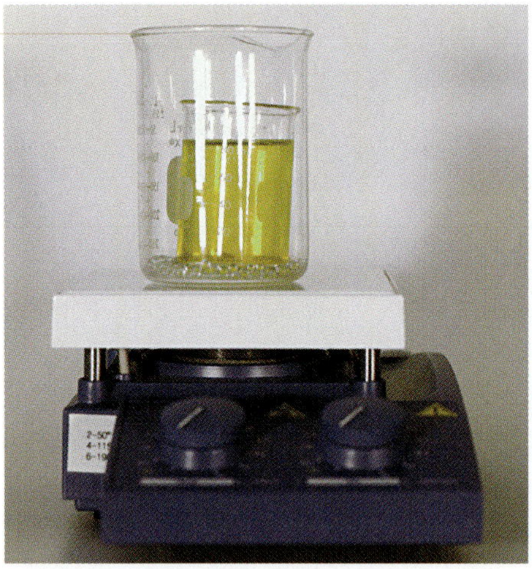

Figure 3-17 Dry bath is an alternative to hotplate and water baths; sand, salt, or aluminum blocks to hold various sizes of glassware

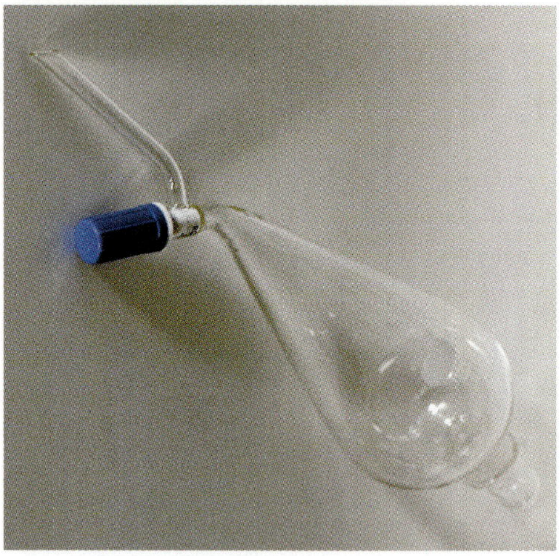

Figure 3-18 Separator

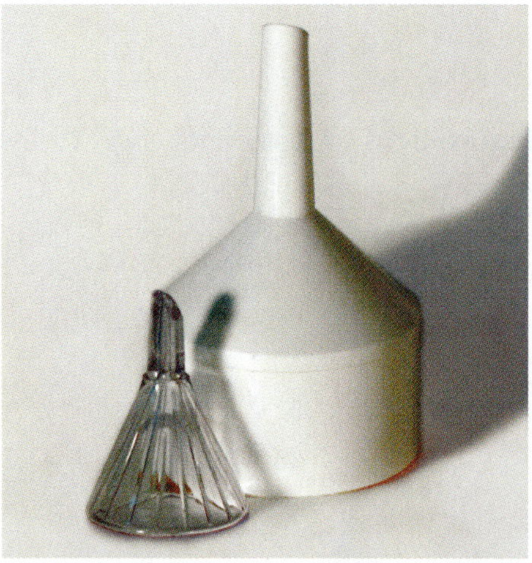

Figure 3-19 Funnels can be glass or plastic and 2", 3", 4", 5", 6"

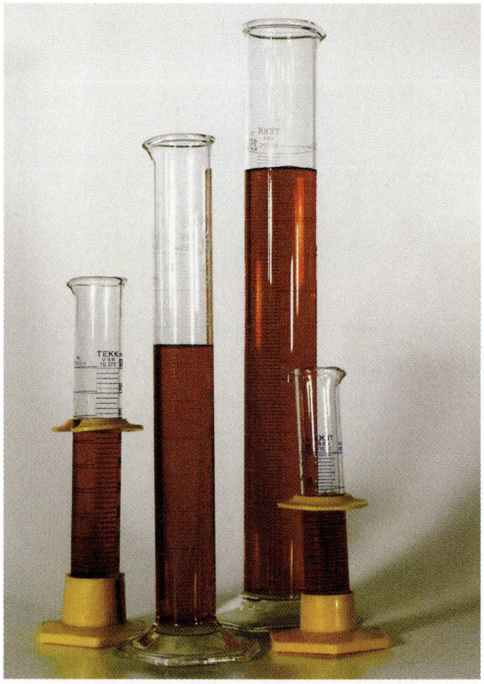

Figure 3-20 Graduates can be pharmaceutical or conical, 10, 25, 50, 100, 250, 500 and 1000 ml, glass or plastic

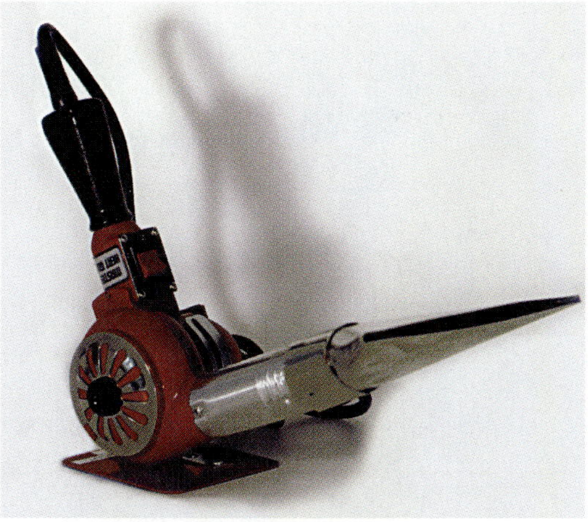

Figure 3-21 Heat gun are used to polish troches, lozenges, and suppositories (also known as a hand-held hair dryer)

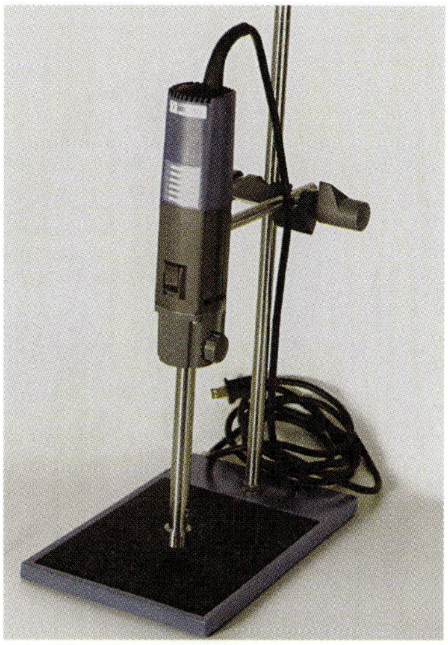

Figure 3-22 Homogenizer is an electronic device used to uniformly suspend particles and reduce particle size

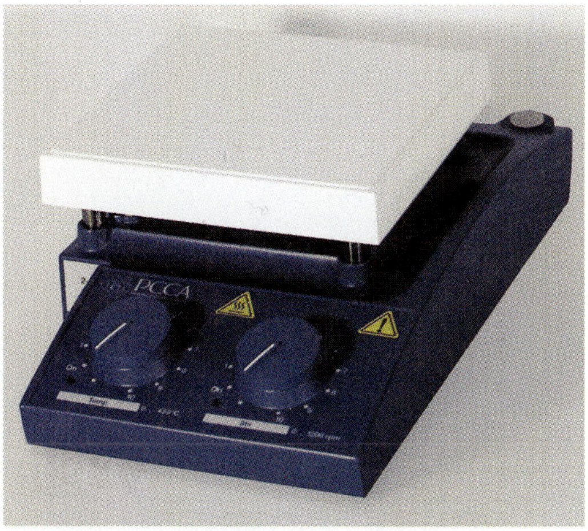

Figure 3-23 Hotplates are available in various sizes with various features

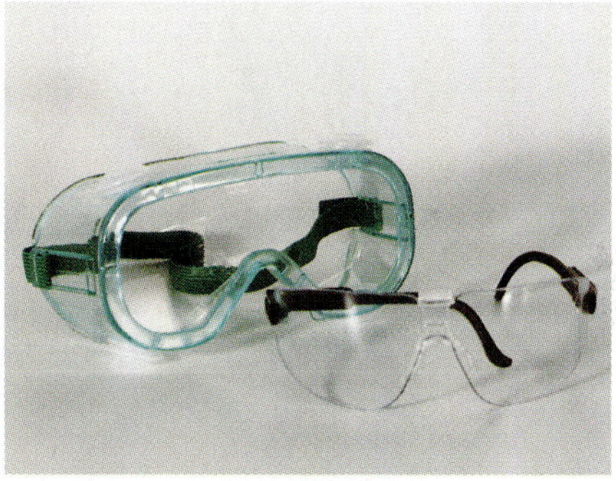

Figure 3-24 Safety glasses

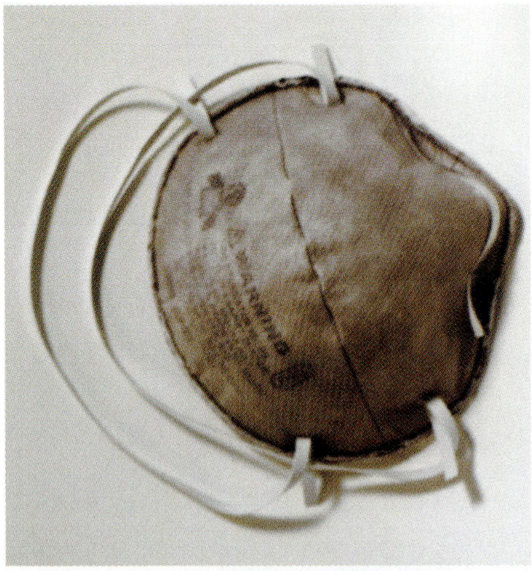

Figure 3-25 A mask protects the preparer from airborne drug particles. Available in various degrees of protection

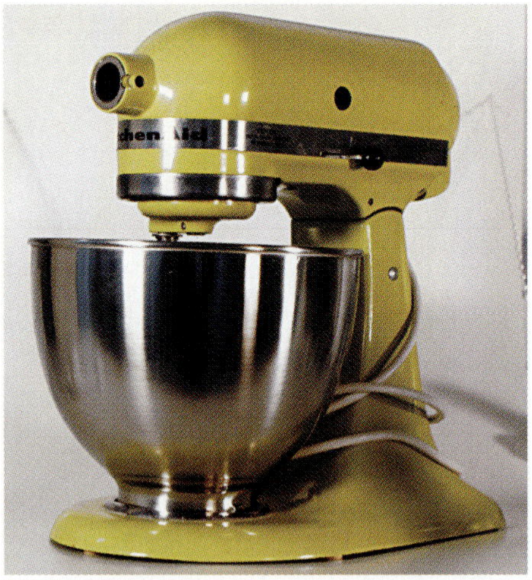

Figure 3-26 A professional mixer, such as a KitchenAid

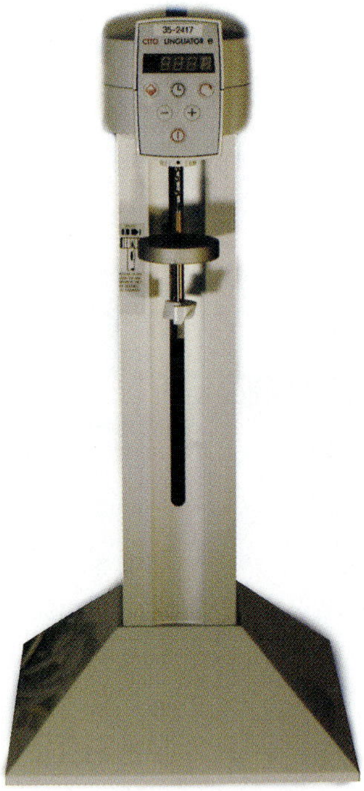

Figure 3-27 Electronic mortar and pestle used for preparing creams, ointments, and gels. Also reduces particle size and uniformly suspends solid ingredients; e.g., Unguator

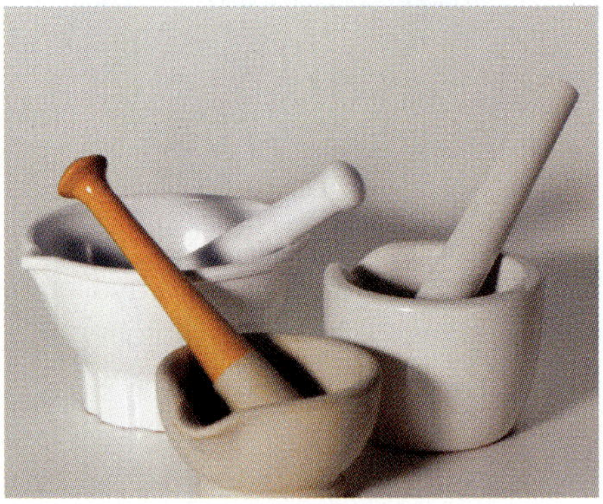

Figure 3-28 Mortars and pestles can be glass, porcelain, or Wedgwood. Size ranges from 1 to 16 oz. Also available in plastic for mixing ointments and creams

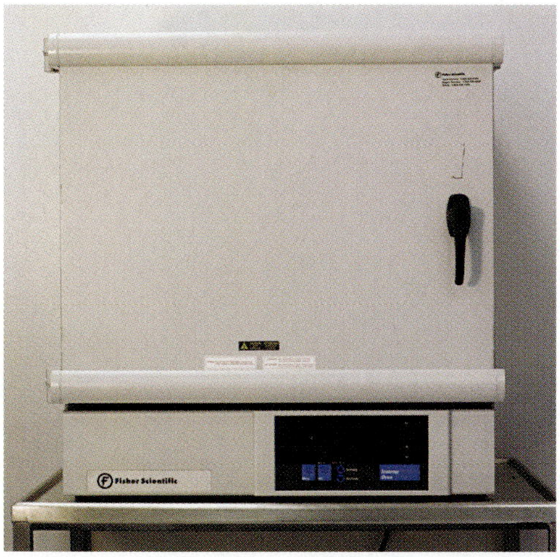

Figure 3-29 Drying oven

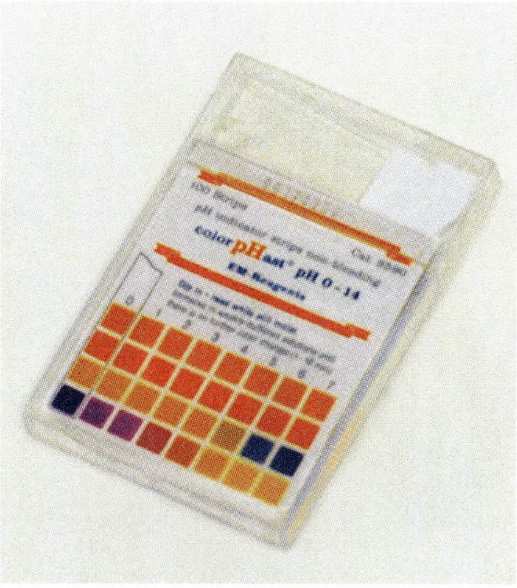

Figure 3-30 pH strips are available in varying degrees of sensitivity and quality

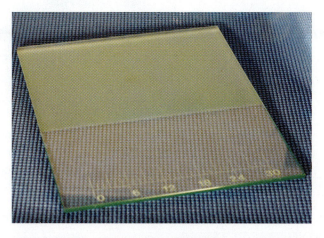

Figure 3-31 Pill tile glass, frosted

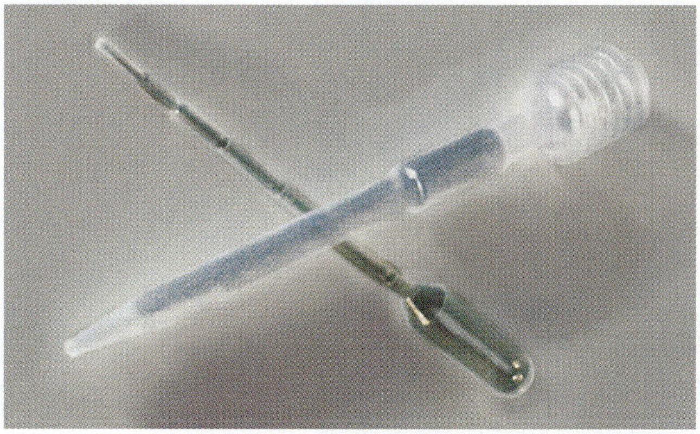

Figure 3-32 Pipettes 1 to 100 ml

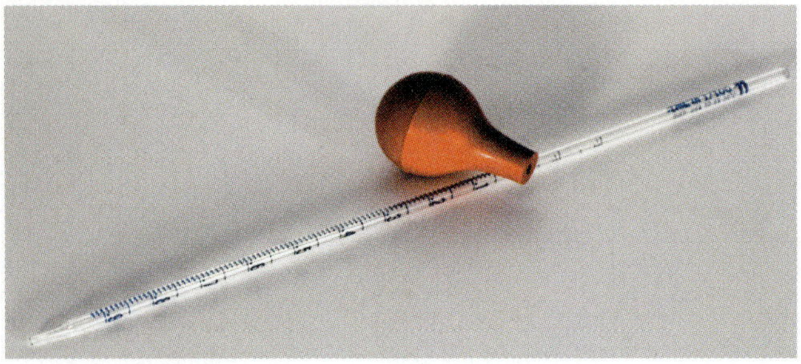

Figure 3-33 Pipette fillers

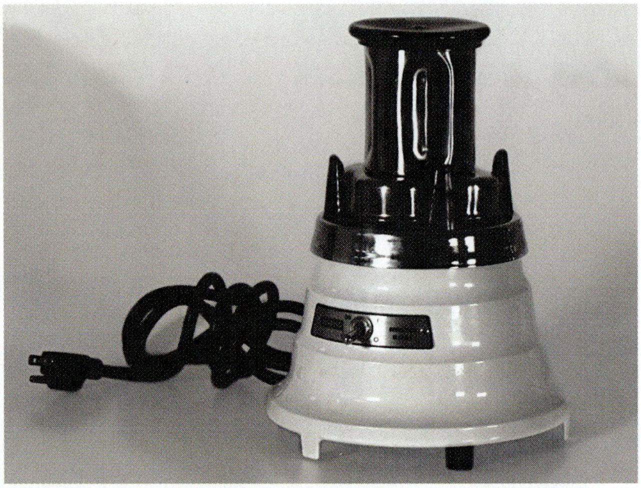

Figure 3-34 Electric powder blender for mixing powders in a dust-free environment, protects the preparer from powder dust. Available in various sizes. Stainless steel

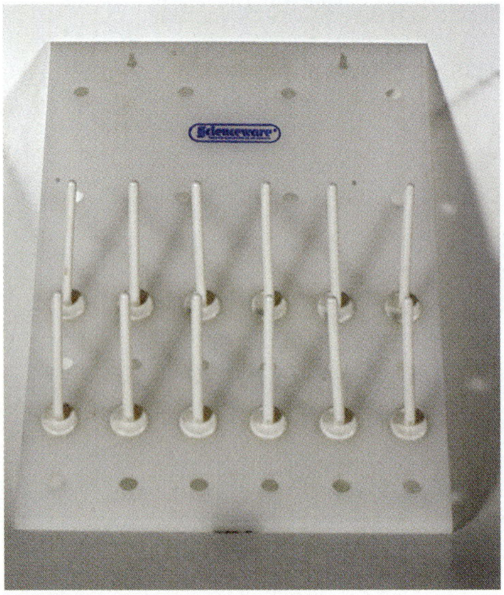

Figure 3-35 Drying rack

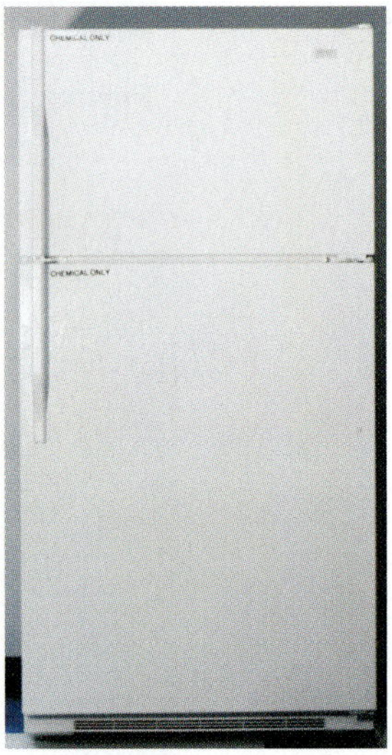

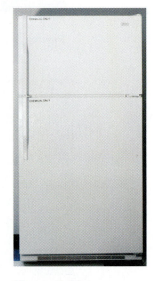

Figure 3-36 Refrigerator with freezer

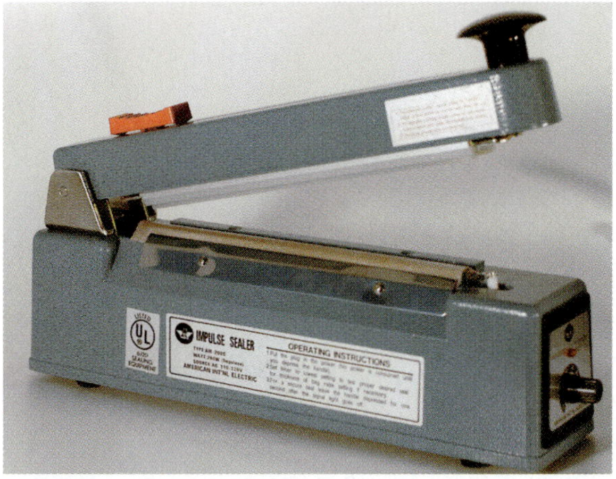

Figure 3-37 Sealer heat, used for sealing tubes or bags

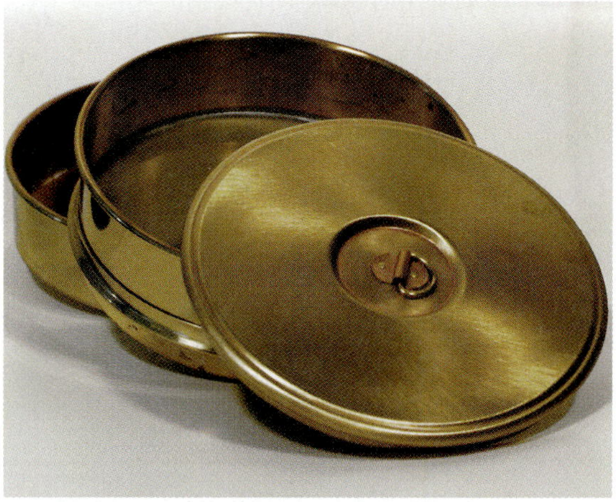

Figure 3-38 Sieve various mesh sizes

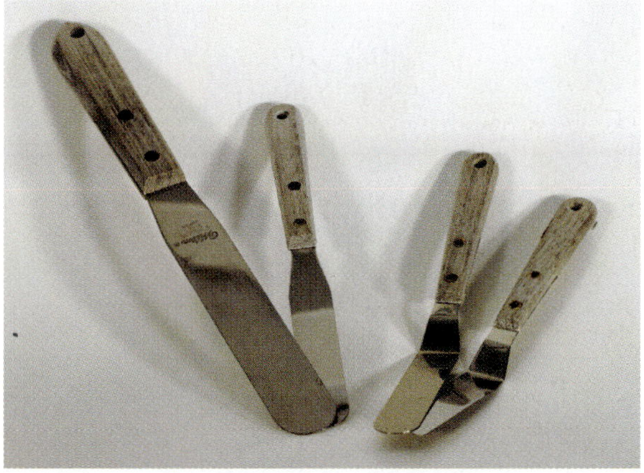

Figure 3-39 Spatulas assorted sizes. Plastic and stainless steel

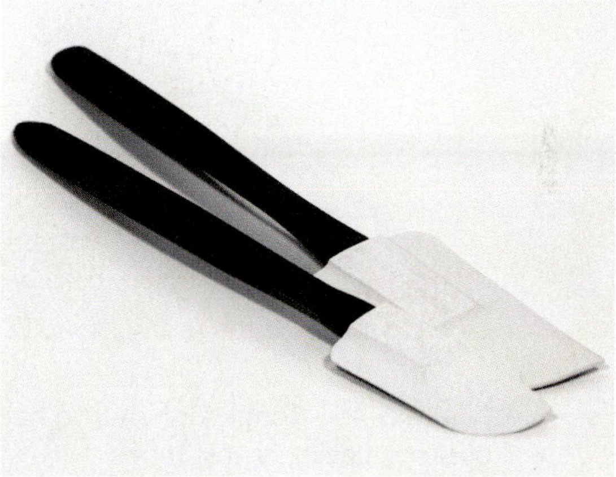

Figure 3-40 Rubber spatulas assorted sizes, kitchen type

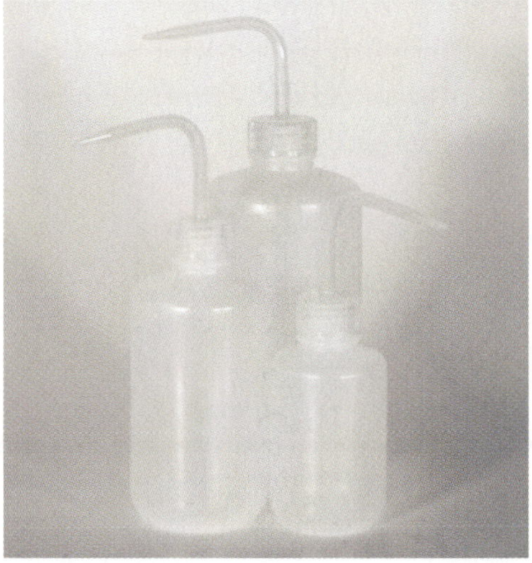

Figure 3-41 Spray bottles

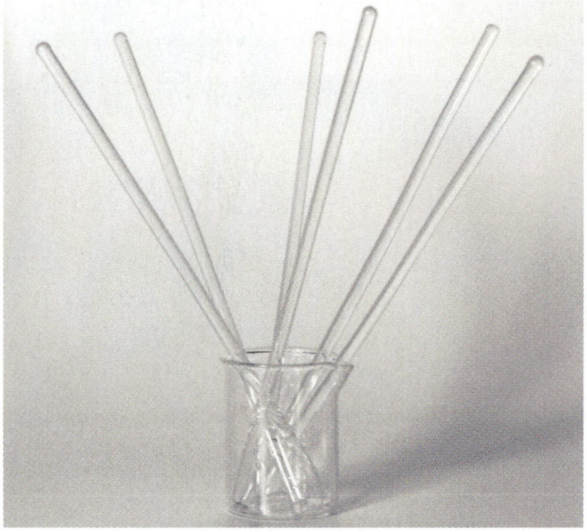

Figure 3-42 Stirring rods

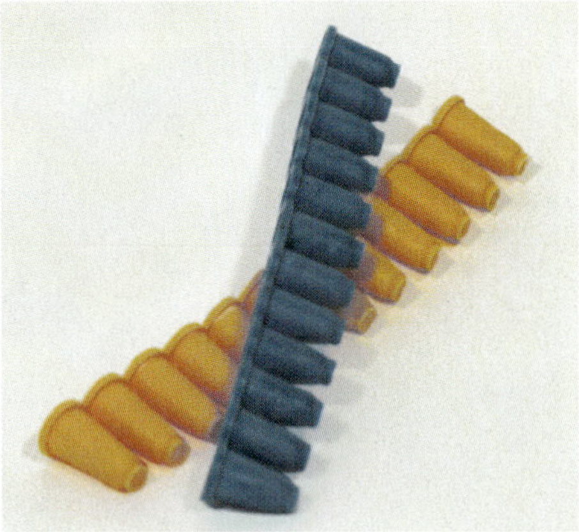

Figure 3-43 Suppository molds rectal, vaginal, and urethral

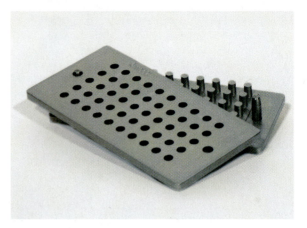

Figure 3-44 Tablet mold for preparing tablets

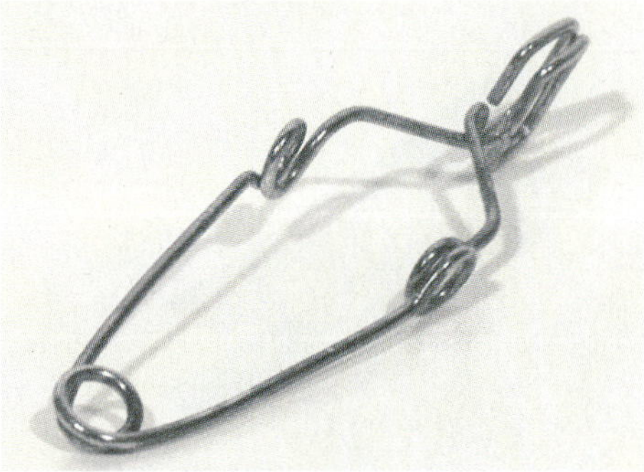

Figure 3-45 Tongs for handling hot beakers, flasks, or test tubes

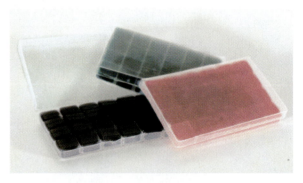

Figure 3-46 Troche molds

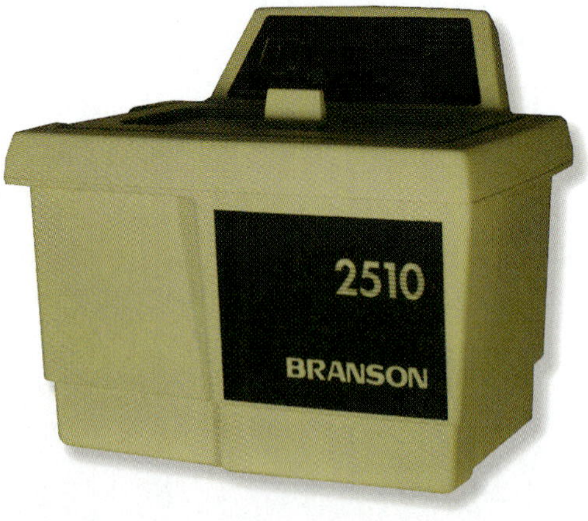

Figure 3-47 Ultrasonic cleaner comes in various capacities

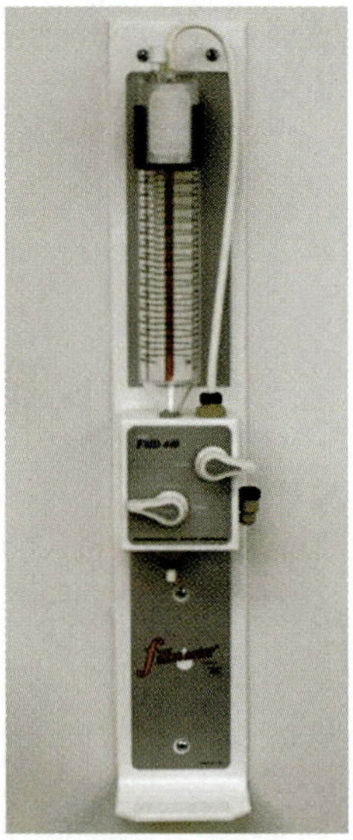

Figure 3-48 Water system

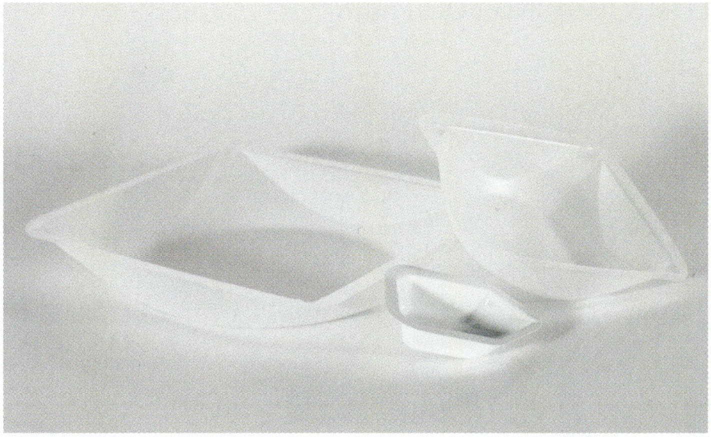

Figure 3-49 Weigh boats come in plastic and various sizes

Figure 3-50 Weigh paper comes in parchment or glacine, and in various sizes

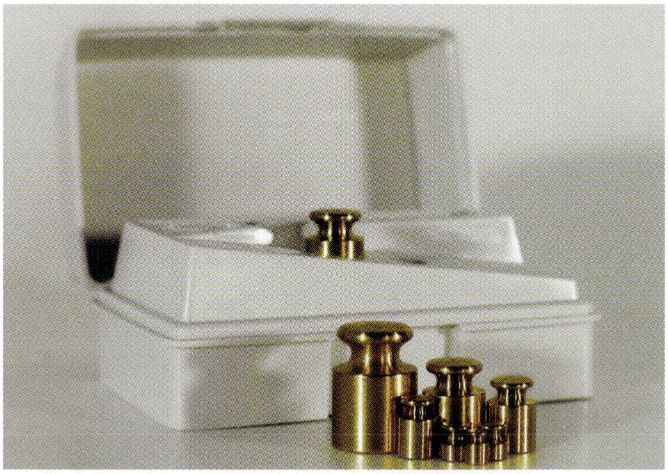

Figure 3-51 Weight sets

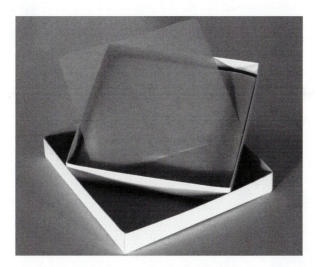

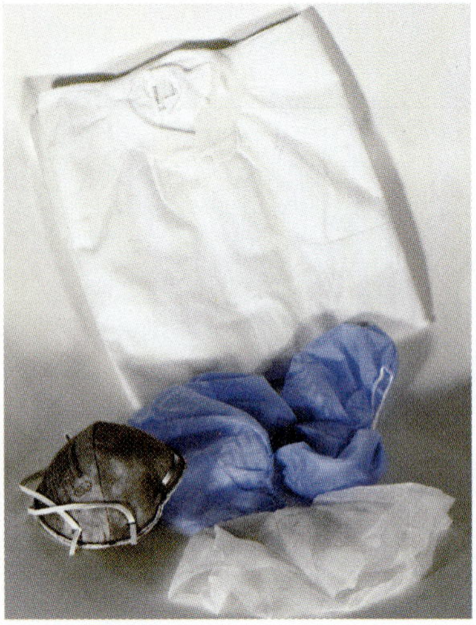

Figure 3-52 Clean room apparel aprons, sleeves, gloves, hoods, boot covers, coveralls, head coverings, lab coats, caps, face masks, beard covers, goggles, etc

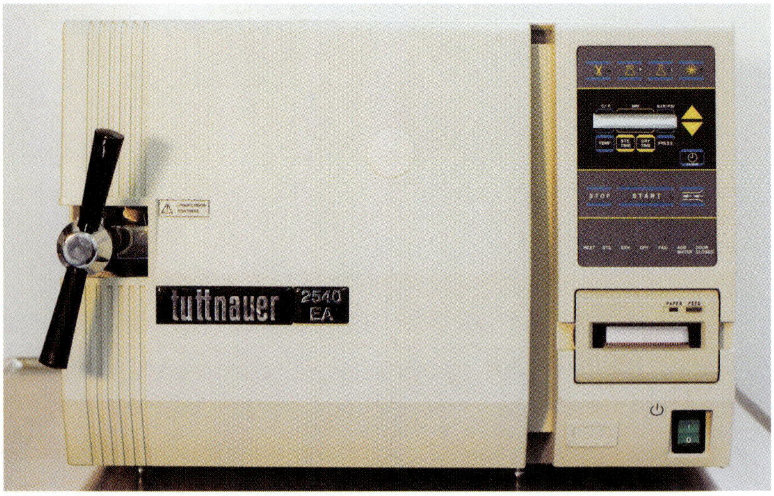

Figure 3-53 Autoclave

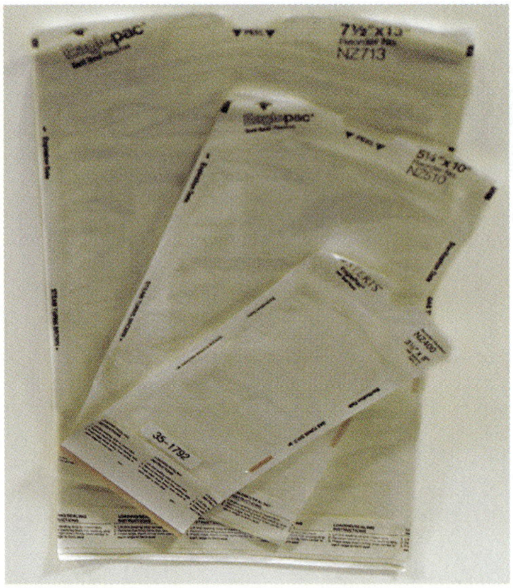

Figure 3-54 Autoclave bags

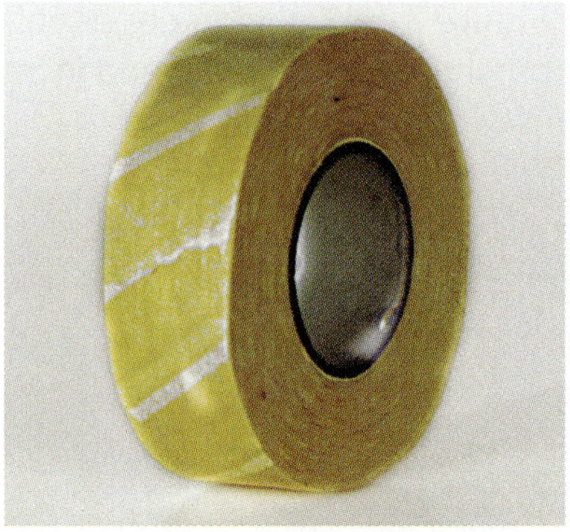

Figure 3-55 Autoclave tape

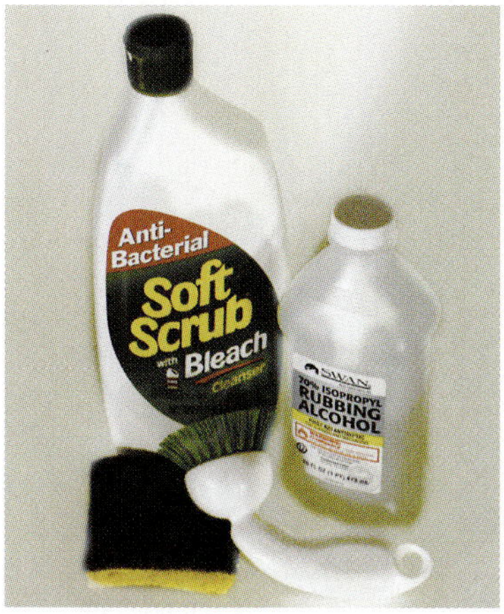

Figure 3-56 Cleaning materials and products

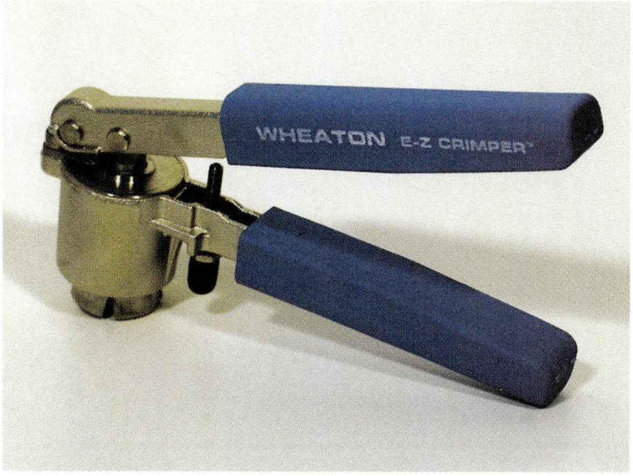

Figure 3-57 Crimper

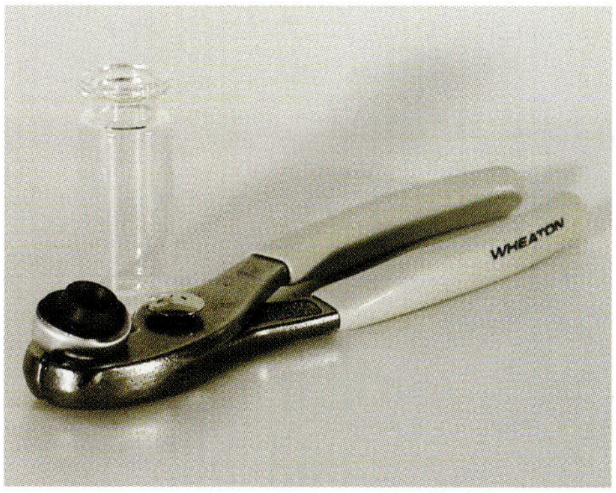

Figure 3-58 Decappers

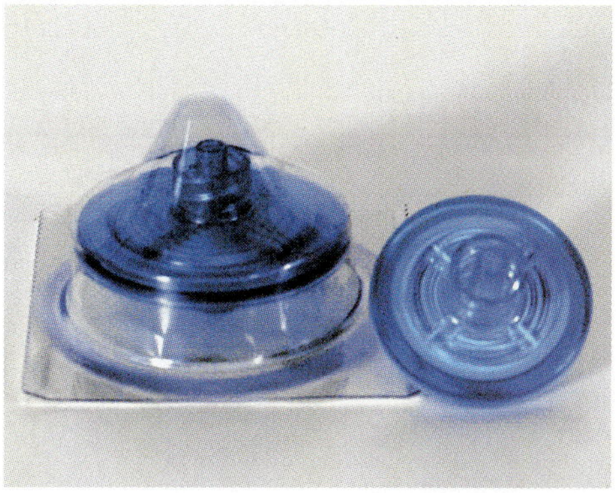

Figure 3-59 Filters numerous types, shapes, applications, and sizes

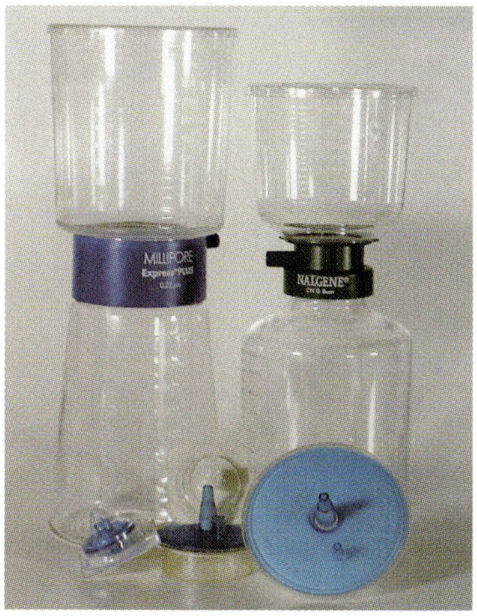

Figure 3-60 Filtration equipment

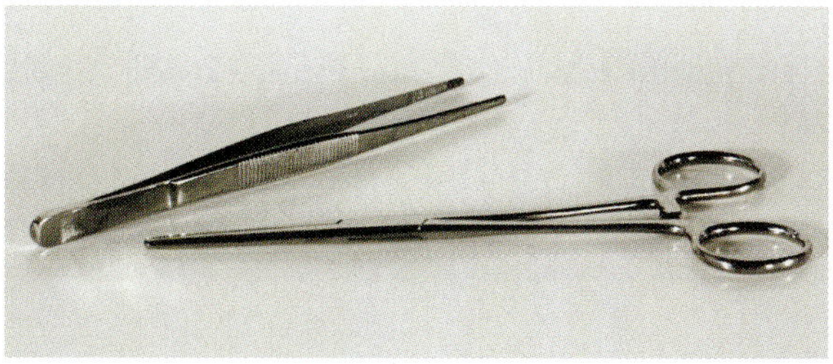

Figure 3-61 Forceps

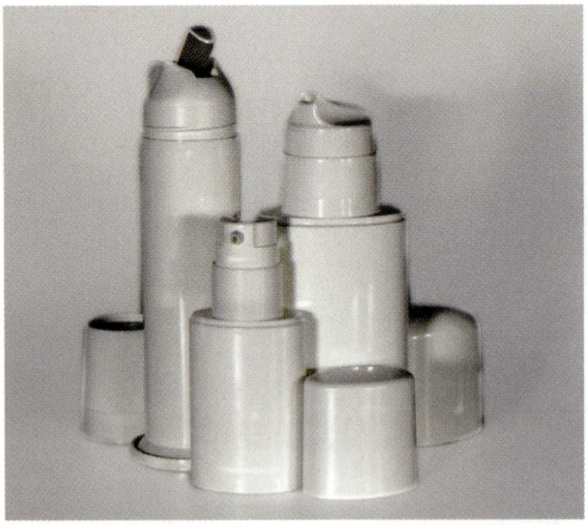

Figure 3-62 Pumps vacuum–Electric, hand operated, or pressure

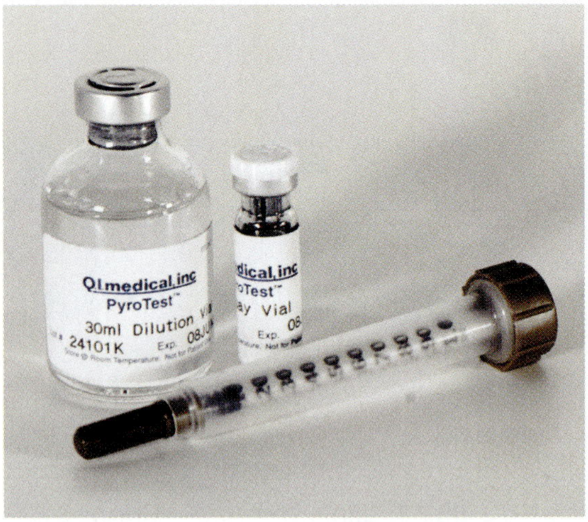

Figure 3-63 Pyrogen test materials

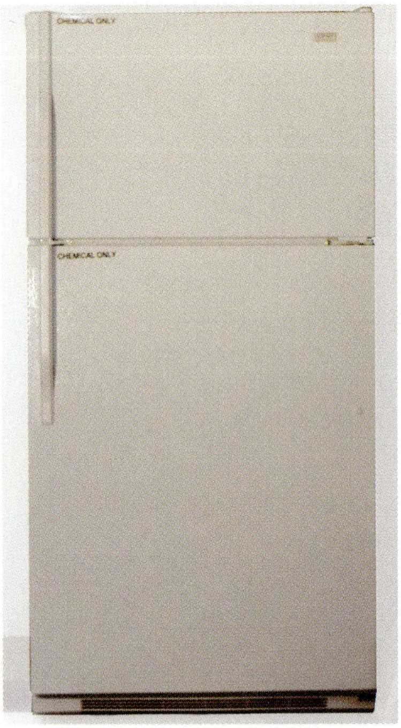

Figure 3-64 Refrigerator with freezer

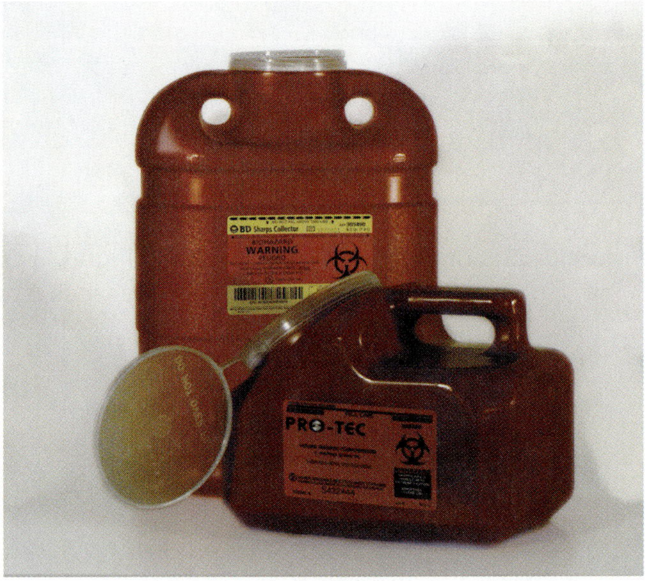

Figure 3-65 Sharps container

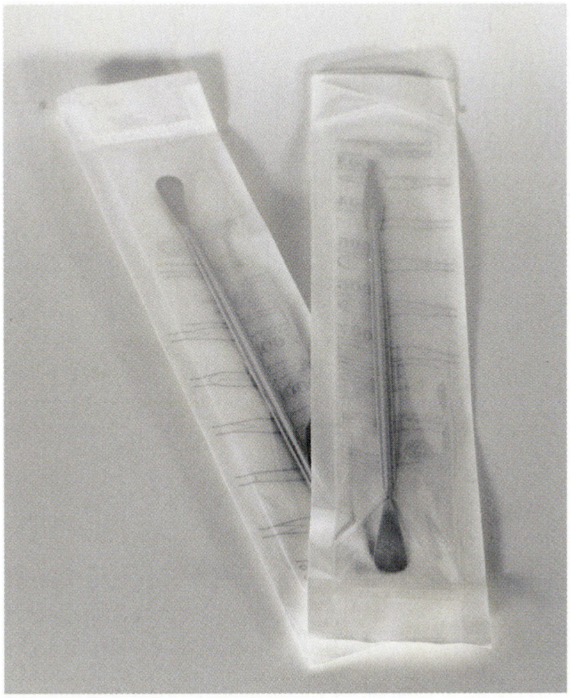

Figure 3-66 Sterile spatulas and spoons

Although this list is comprehensive, it is certainly not complete. Each day presents the compounding pharmacy with new challenges. As these challenges are presented, solutions must be obtained. With each solution comes the problem of making the idea work. In order to make the idea work, a unique tool may be necessary to accomplish the task. Thus, new tools are being developed almost daily. Tools used in compounding can be anything but traditional. A good compounding technician will be creative in finding working solutions and coming up with tools to attempt the idea.

SUMMARY

While every compounding pharmacy is individual and unique, there are standard facilities, equipment, and supplies they all need. Proper tools that have been well-maintained, quality supplies that are easy to locate, and a workspace that is clean and organized are all essential to compounding.

CHAPTER TERMS

cross-contamination
when bacteria or particulates migrate to an undesired space and have the potential to cause harm.

distilled water
the most common diluent used in compounding.

isopropyl 70 percent alcohol
an acceptable substance used to wipe down areas to help keep them as clean as possible.

SOP
Standard Operating Procedure, a documentation of the operation of a process.

work station
the area defined inside a clean room where the compounding takes place.

CHAPTER 3

CHAPTER REVIEW QUESTIONS

1. The following are the main considerations when setting up a compounding laboratory, *excluding*
   a. facilities
   b. marketing
   c. equipment
   d. supplies

2. How often should the compounding laboratory be thoroughly cleaned?
   a. every one to seven days
   b. every two weeks
   c. every month
   d. twice daily

3. If a station for preparing liquid medications is set up, which of the following items should be stored in that area?
   a. gelatin capsules
   b. crimper
   c. foil wraps
   d. adaptacaps

4. How should glassware, such as mortars and pestles or graduates and beakers, be stored?
   a. in cabinets with doors, turned upside down
   b. in cabinets with doors, turned right side up
   c. on shelves, turned upside down
   d. on shelves, turned right side up

5. Which of the following is an electronic device used to uniformly suspend particles and reduce particle size?
   a. centrifuge
   b. desiccator
   c. homogenizer
   d. autoclave

6. True or false: Easy work flow and cleanliness are the most important characteristics of a compounding facility or compounding area.
   a. true
   b. false

7. True or false: Contaminated clothing, gloves, masks, and trash from the compounding procedure should be disposed of with the other pharmacy trash.
   a. true
   b. false

8. List five pieces of equipment used in nonsterile compounding.

9. Where should a compounding area within an existing pharmacy setting be established?

10. **Critical Thinking** Draw a floorplan for a pharmacy that compounds liquids, creams, molds, and capsules. Label each item on the floorplan and provide a written description, which includes the reason for your design.

Resources and References

1. Allen, Loyd V. Jr., Ph.D. *The Art, Science, and Technology of Pharmaceutical Compounding*. Washington, DC: American Pharmaceutical Association, 1998.
2. Allen, Loyd V. Jr., Ph.D. *Secundum Artem: Pharmacy Compounding Equipment*. Minneapolis, MN: Paddock Laboratories.

CHAPTER 4

Quality Assurance and Record Keeping

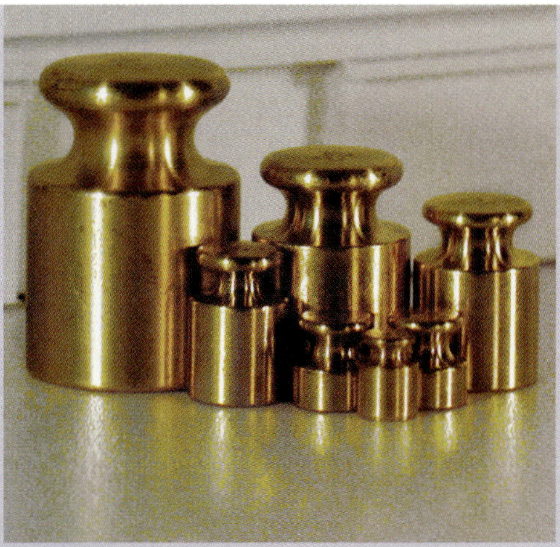

Learning Objectives

After completing this chapter, you should be able to:

- Define quality control and quality assurance.
- Recognize standard operating procedures (SOPs) and how to use them.
- Explain how to perform end-product testing on non-sterile compounds.
- Explain how to perform end-product testing on sterile compounds.
- List the records required for compounding activities.
- To properly document information about compounding activities.
- Describe the proper training required of compounding personnel.

INTRODUCTION

Commercially available medications are manufactured by pharmaceutical companies. All of these commercial products must meet certain standards of quality and pass all of the end-product testing set by the industry standards and the **FDA**. The standards are established to ensure that patients and consumers receive safe and effective products.

On the other hand, compounding is regulated by the state boards of pharmacy and the U.S. Pharmacopeia. Most state boards of pharmacy recognize the U.S. Pharmacopeia as the standard for pharmacy practice, and all of the chapters under 1000 are legally enforceable. Compounding is also legally recognized by the Federal Food, Drug, and Cosmetic Act. This Act was a 1997 amendment to the Food and Drug Administration Modernization Act to protect the pharmacists' right to compound, provided that all compounding is conducted within specific parameters, especially maintaining the **triad** relationship.

Although compounded products are prepared on an individual basis to meet the special needs of a patient or patient population, the pharmacy should have a good quality assurance program and maintain proper records to ensure that the patient is receiving a safe, stable, and properly compounded medication.

FDA
Food and Drug Administration

triad
the professional relationship between the pharmacist, patient, and physician

audit
an examination of records to verify accuracy

pyrogenicity
producing or produced by fever

calibration
the set of gradients that show position or value

Quality Assurance (QA)

Quality assurance is a program of activities used to ensure that the procedures used in the preparation of compounded products lead to products that meet certain specifications and standards. A good quality assurance program should include the following:

- Documented, ongoing QA program for training, monitoring, and evaluating pharmacy personnel performance.
- Documented, ongoing QA program for testing and monitoring equipment used in compounding.
- Documented, ongoing QA program for monitoring and testing compounded products.
- Documented, ongoing QA program for monitoring and evaluating patient outcomes to ensure efficacy of the compounded products.
- Written plan for corrective action if problems are identified by the QA **audits** or testing.
- Documented periodic review of the QA activities for effectiveness.

Quality Control (QC)

Quality control is a set of testing activities used to determine the quality of the compounded products. The testing focuses on the ingredients, devices or components, and the final products prepared to determine if they meet required standards of identity and purity. Sterile products must also meet sterility and **pyrogenicity** standards. In general, quality control is the daily control or management of quality within the pharmacy. Quality control should include the following:

- *Standard operating procedures (SOPs)* to document the **calibration** and maintenance of equipment used in compounding.
- SOPs to document pharmacy personnel initial and ongoing training and validation.
- SOP for product recalls.
- SOP to document monitoring of the compounding environment, both sterile and nonsterile.
- SOPs to evaluate, confirm, and document the quality of the final compounded products.

Records and Record Keeping

Record keeping is an essential component of every quality assurance program and quality control. Good record keeping accomplishes the following:

- Provides information about each ingredient in a compounded product.
- Facilitates a product recall, if necessary.
- Enables pharmacy personnel to consistently duplicate a compounded product or testing procedure.
- Provides information about QC testing procedures and equipment.

There are five types of records that should be maintained in a compounding pharmacy:

- SOPs with sign-off or log sheets.
- Formulation records or "recipe" sheets.
- Compounding records for each compound prepared.
- Ingredient records that include Certificates of Analysis and Material Safety Data Sheets (MSDSs).
- Equipment maintenance records.

Records may be kept manually as hard copies or electronically, using computer software programs. Both manual and electronic systems have advantages and disadvantages, although keeping both types of records is preferred. Hard copies can be filed in a cabinet or kept in notebooks. They are readily available when computer systems fail. In a manual system, however, it may be difficult to obtain specific information, such as all of the compounds that used a specific ingredient which has been recalled. When changes are made in an SOP or formulation with a manual system, the entire record will need to be redone. Electronic records are readily available and easy to modify, and specific information can be quickly retrieved when there is an ingredient recall. Electronic systems can generate all of the necessary forms and labels, and keep track of inventories and all compounding activities.

Standard Operating Procedures (SOPs)

A standard operating procedure (SOP) is a set of step-by-step written instructions on how to do a certain task. All important tasks performed in a compounding pharmacy should be covered by SOPs and documentation. SOPs should be developed for facility maintenance; equipment calibration and maintenance; personnel training and validation; and the preparation, packaging, and storage of compounded items. SOPs should also include sign-off or log sheets to document that the SOPs have been followed.

SOPs are necessary because there may be more than one way to do a particular task. For example, each technician or pharmacist may clean the clean room in a different manner. One person may prefer to clean all of the shelving and countertops with 70 percent isopropyl alcohol, while another person would clean the area weekly with a different type of disinfectant. An SOP for this task would clearly define, step by step, how to consistently perform this routine task and possibly prevent bacterial resistance by using the same **disinfectant** all of the time.

disinfectant
an agent or a chemical that destroys, neutralizes, or inhibits the growth of disease-carrying microorganisms

There is a common saying, "If it has not been documented, it was never done." All tasks completed need to be documented on a sign-off or log sheet. If a problem arises with the task, the logs or records may provide information that can be used to correct the problem.
SOPs can assure that

- The equipment is properly maintained and calibrated.
- Supplies and chemicals are received, inventoried, compliant with compounding standards, stored properly, and disposed of correctly.
- All procedures and tasks are performed consistently and documented.

Since SOPs require logs and sign-off sheets to maintain proper records, a notebook or file should be kept for each SOP to organize and maintain these records for easy retrieval. Depending on the pharmacy or organization, SOPs generally follow a uniform format:

1. SOP number—a unique number assigned to distinguish between SOPs.
2. Date effective—the date that the SOP is implemented.
3. Author—the name of the person who wrote the SOP.
4. Authorization signature—signature of the pharmacy administrator who approves the SOP.
5. Purpose of procedure—one or two brief sentences explaining why the task or procedure is being done.
6. Equipment/Materials—list of equipment or materials needed to perform the SOP.
7. Procedure—a detailed step-by-step explanation that can be easily followed by different individuals to obtain the same results.
8. Documentation forms—sheets that record the results of the SOP. The information documented should include the date that the SOP is performed, the operator's signature, and the results. A comment line is optional, but can be used to explain and document unusual results.

Figure 4-1 is an example of an SOP used to monitor air temperature.

Figure 4-2 is an example of the log that should be kept in a notebook to document that this SOP is being properly done.

WORKPLACE WISDOM

The formulation record is commonly referred to as the "recipes."

Formulation Records

Formulation records are specific step-by-step instructions on how to prepare the compound. These records may be kept and maintained as hard copies in a book or in file folders. They also may be filed electronically, using a commercially available software program.

Compounding is not an exact science, and there may be more than one way to make a particular product. For example, metronidazole 50 mg/ml suspension may be prepared by two different methods: crushing tablets into a powder or using metronidazole benzoate powder, USP. See Table 4-1.

Both methods result in a 50 mg/ml metronidazole suspension, but the final products are vastly different. The formulation using the tablets may be thicker because of the excipients in the tablets. This formulation also is not very **palatable**, because the tablets contain metronidazole base, which has a very bitter taste. The formulation using the powder may be thinner because

palatable
acceptable to the taste

Figure 4-1 Sample SOP

Standard Operating Procedures

SOP #________

Date Effective:

Revision Number:

Person Preparing:

Person Checking:

Purpose of Procedure:

[The purpose of the procedure should be described.]

Procedure:

[The procedure should be detailed in a step-by-step fashion so that it can be easily followed by different individuals with the same results. It should contain sufficient detail and descriptive information to minimize any required interpretation.]

1.

2.

3.

4.

5.

Documentation Forms:

[The results of the standard operating procedure may need to be documented onto a form and maintained in a notebook for easy retrieval. In this case, the organization of the forms notebook should parallel that of the SOP notebook. The reference point can be the SOP number, which should be placed on each page. Space should be available for a description of the procedure that was done, date, operator's signature, and the results.]

there are no extra excipients. This formulation uses a different salt form of metronidazole, benzoate instead of base, which has very little taste, and the OraSweet® makes it taste good. The method of preparation may also affect the stability of the compound. Unknown excipients in tablets may make the compound less stable, and the patient may need to get refills more often.

Figure 4-2 Sample SOP compliance log

Temperature Log for ABC Pharmacy

Month / Year: ____________________________

Date	Refrigerator Temperature	Room Temperature	Initials
1			
2			
3			
4			
5			
6			
7			
8			
9			
10			
11			
12			
13			
14			
15			
16			
17			
18			
19			
20			
21			
22			
23			
24			
25			
26			
27			
28			
29			
30			
31			

The formulation record ensures that the compound will be prepared by the pharmacy personnel in a consistent manner. It should include the following information:

- Name, strength, and dosage form of the preparation.
- All ingredients and their quantities.
- Equipment required to compound the preparation.
- Pertinent calculations.

Table 4-1 Comparison of Compounding Procedures to Prepare Metronidazole 50 mg/ml Suspension

Procedure Using Tablets[1]	Procedure Using Benzoate Powder[2]
1. Grind 24 metronidazole 250 mg tablets into a powder in a mortar with pestle.	1. Weigh 8 gm metronidazole benzoate powder and place in a mortar.
2. Levigate with a small amount of a 1 : 1 mixture of Ora-Sweet® and Ora-Plus® to form a paste.	2. Wet the powder with a small amount of glycerin and mix into a thick paste.
3. Add the Ora-Sweet® and Ora-Plus® base in increasing amounts while mixing thoroughly.	3. Pour a portion of a 1 : 1 mixture of Ora Sweet® and Ora-Plus® base until wetted powder is evenly suspended.
4. Pour contents into a graduated cylinder.	4. Pour mixture into a graduated cylinder.
5. QS to the desired volume.	5. QS to the desired volume.
6. Pour the mixture into a clean prescription bottle, cap, and shake well to mix.	6. Pour the mixture into a clean prescription bottle, cap, and shake well to mix.
7. Seal and label.	7. Seal and label.

[1]Allen L.V. Jr., Erickson III, M.A. "Stability of ketoconazole, metolazone, metronidazole, procainamide hydrochloride, and spironolactone in extemporaneously compounded oral liquids." *American Journal of Health System Pharmacy*. 1996 Sep. 1; 53(17): 2073–8.
[2]Matthew, M., Gupta, V.D., Bethea, C. The development of oral liquid dosage forms of metronidazole. *J Clin Pharm Ther*. Vol. 19, 1994. pp. 27–29.

- Step-by-step mixing instructions.
- QC procedures.
- Reference citation(s).
- Beyond-use date or expiration date.
- Container(s) or devices used.
- Storage requirements.

Figure 4-3 is an example of formulation record format.

Compounding Records

The compounding record is the written documentation for the preparation of the compounded product. The formulation record, or "recipe," can be modified to also become the compounding record, or "worksheet" (Figure 4-4).

The following information should be included on the worksheet:

- Formulation record used for the product.
- Information about each ingredient (including quantity, measured or weighed), manufacturer, manufacturer's lot number, and manufacturer's expiration date.
- Quantity of product prepared (in ml, grams, or number of units prepared).
- Signature of pharmacist or technician compounding the product.
- Signature or initials of pharmacist doing final or double checks.
- Date of preparation.
- Assigned lot number and/or prescription number.
- QC testing results.

WORKPLACE WISDOM

The compounding record is commonly referred to as the "worksheet."

Figure 4-3 Sample formulation record "Recipe"

Compound Name

SUGGESTED FORMULA FOR

#1 Capsules - Per Capsules

Active Ingredient: .... 50 milligrams

Inactive Ingredient: .... 400 milligrams

SUGGESTED COMPOUNDING PROCEDURE

1. Step by step
2. Step by step

WARNING!
SAFETY WHEN COMPOUNDING

Precaution .... Precaution .... Precaution ....

In retail settings, it is common for pharmacy personnel to document, on the actual prescription label, only the date that a compound was prepared and the pharmacist's initials. There is minimal compounding information documented on the prescription. This is not an adequate compounding record. All pharmacies, in both retail and hospital settings, should keep thorough compounding records to ensure the quality and consistency of the compounded product. Proper documentation may also help protect the pharmacy legally if the compounded product is involved in an adverse event.

COMPOUNDING FORMULA WORKSHEET

Name of Drug: ____________ **Description:** ____________ **Compounding NDC# (if applicable):** ____________

Time to Make: ______ **minutes** **Code:** ______ **Schedule:** ______ **Therapy:** ______ **Misc:** ______

Days to Expire: ______

Name of Drug	Form	Obtained From Supplier	Manufacturer & NDC #	Lot # and Expiration	Amount Needed Per Unit	Total Units to Make	Total Volume Required	Made By	RPh

Instructions/Notes:

1. ______
2. ______
3. ______
4. ______
5. ______
6. ______

Date Made: ______ Lot #: ______ Expiration Date: ______

Quantity Made: ______ Made By: ______

Final Check By: ______

ABC PHARMACY

Quality Control

BATCH TEST: 1. Unit Weight ______ **Total Weight** ______
BATCH TEST: 2. Unit Weight ______ **Total Weight** ______
BATCH TEST: 3. Unit Weight ______ **Total Weight** ______
BATCH TEST: 4. Unit Weight ______ **Total Weight** ______

Any variations in testing? YES or NO **Follow up required? YES or NO** **If follow up, what procedure was done?** ______

Was drug released for dispensing? YES or NO **If not released, what procedure was followed?** ______

Figure 4-4 Sample compounding record "Worksheet"

Ingredient Records

Chemicals should be USP or NF quality, and the pharmacy should maintain records of all the chemicals purchased, including Certificates of Analysis. These certificates are issued by the chemical wholesalers and are proof of the chemicals' purity. Commercially available finished products do not require certificates of analysis.

Material Safety Data Sheets (MSDSs) contain the following information about the chemicals:

- Physiochemical information.
- Toxicity information, including precautions and potential hazards.
- Handling information, including disposal.
- Shipping instructions, including required labeling.

All pharmacy personnel should review the information to protect themselves, as well as the patient. Everyone should be instructed on the location of the MSDSs. These records should be kept on file as original hard copies. MSDSs are free and commonly shipped with bulk chemicals from the wholesalers. They are also easily obtained from the Internet. (See Figure 4-5.)

MSDS

NAME: Specific Drug
CAS #: 57-85-2
MF: C22H3203

Synonyms:

TOXICITY HAZARDS

Rtecs No: ____________________

Figure 4-5 Sample MSDS

Toxicity Data:

Reviews, standards, and regulations:

Target organ data:

HEALTH HAZARD DATA

Acute effects:

Chronic effects:

First aid:

PHYSICAL DATA

Melting pt: 122 C to 123
Appearance and odor: white powder

FIRE AND EXPLOSION HAZARD DATA

Extinguishing media:

Special firefighting procedures:

Figure 4-5 Sample MSDS (*continued*)

Unusual fire and explosions hazards:

REACTIVITY DATA

Stability: Stable.

Incompatibilities:
Strong oxidizing agents, strong bases

Hazardous combustion or decomposition products toxic fumes of:
Carbon monoxide, carbon dioxide.

Hazardous polymerization will not occur.

SPILL OR LEAK PROCEDURE

Steps to be taken if material is released or spilled:
Evacuate area. Wear self-contained breathing apparatus, rubber boots and heavy rubber gloves. Wear disposable coveralls and discard them after use. Sweep up, place in a bag and hold for waste disposal. Ventilate area and wash spill site after material pickup is complete.

Waste disposal method:
Contact the drug enforcement administration concerning the disposal of controlled substances. Observe all federal, state, and local laws.

PRECAUTIONS TO BE TAKEN IN HANDLING AND STORAGE

Wear appropriate NIOSH/MSHA-approved respirator, chemical-resistant gloves, safety goggles, other protective clothing. Use only in a chemical fume hood. Safety shower and eye bath. May cause cancer. Harmful by inhalation, in contact with skin and if swallowed. possible risk of irreversible effects. If you feel unwell, seek medical advice (show the label where possible). Wear suitable protective clothing, gloves, and eye/face protection. Keep container tightly closed in a cool well ventilated place. Possible teratogen.

The above information on this MSDS was obtained from current and reputable sources. However the data is provided without warranty, expressed or implied, regardless of its correctness or accuracy. It is the user's responsibility both to determine safe conditions for use of this product and to assume liability for loss, injury, damage or expense resulting from improper use of this product.

Figure 4-5 Sample MSDS (*continued*)

Training Personnel

The pharmacist is responsible for all compounding activities, including ensuring that the technicians are well trained and receive ongoing training. Trained pharmacists and technicians understand the importance of each task or SOP and are efficient, safe, and motivated.

All compounding pharmacy personnel should read and understand all of the SOPs and compounding guidelines, including Chapter (795), "Pharmacy Compounding," of the *United States Pharmacopeia 25/National Formulary 20 (USP 25/NF 20)* and Chapter (797), "Sterile Compounding," of the *United States Pharmacopeia 27/National Formulary 22 (USP 27/NF 22)*. Technicians should receive hands-on, step-by-step training in all SOPs and compounding techniques. When a technician can demonstrate to the pharmacist a verbal and operational knowledge of each SOP, the pharmacist should document, on a log sheet, that the training has been completed and should keep the log sheet on file. Certificates from formal training programs in compounding should also be kept on file.

Most chemical wholesalers and some companies that manufacture compounding products offer formal, accredited training programs in various aspects of compounding: comprehensive (general overview), sterile compounding, veterinary compounding, hormone replacement therapy (HRT), and pain management. Employers usually pay part or all of the expenses for pharmacists and technicians to attend these classes. Ongoing training and continuing education (CE) programs can be obtained through compounding publications, such as *Secundum Artem* and the *International Journal of Pharmaceutical Compounding*, as well as on-the-job reviews and training on new SOPs implemented.

When there is a question about compounding, a pharmacy technician should ask the supervising pharmacist to answer it. A lack of understanding of an SOP could result in a substandard compounded product, loss of labor time, or potential harm to the patient.

SUMMARY

Compounding pharmacies are held to specific standards for quality, similar to federal standards imposed on pharmaceutical manufacturers. These standards on quality assurance and quality control provide parameters for individual pharmacies to safely and effectively compound medications for specific patient needs.

CHAPTER TERMS

audit
an examination of records to verify accuracy

calibration
the set of gradients that show position or value

disinfectant
an agent or a chemical that destroys, neutralizes, or inhibits the growth of disease-carrying microorganisms

FDA
Food and Drug Administration

palatable
acceptable to the taste

pyrogenicity
producing or produced by fever

triad
the professional relationship between the pharmacist, patient, and physician

CHAPTER 4

CHAPTER REVIEW QUESTIONS

1. Compounded products must meet certain standards of quality and pass all of the end-product testing set by the industry standards and which of the following?

   a. DEA
   b. ASHP
   c. FDA
   d. ATF

2. A detailed step-by-step explanation that can be easily followed by different individuals to obtain the same results is known as

   a. a QA report
   b. a requisition
   c. a C12-131 Form
   d. an SOP

3. What is the term for a set of testing activities used to determine the quality of the compounded products?

   a. quality assurance
   b. quality control
   c. an SOP
   d. formulation

4. Fill in the blank: Chemicals should be _____ or _____ quality.

   a. USP or NF
   b. FDA or DEA
   c. clean or pure
   d. chemical or food

5. What ensures that the compound will be prepared by the pharmacy personnel in a consistent manner?

   a. the SOP
   b. the formulation record
   c. the quality assurance worksheet
   d. the quality control report

6. True or False: Records may be kept electronically utilizing computer software.

   a. true
   b. false

7. True or false: The common saying regarding quality assurance and record keeping is "If it has not been documented, then it cannot be audited."

   a. true
   b. false

8. What is the purpose of an SOP?

9. List three out of the five types of records that should be maintained in a compounding pharmacy.

10. Look back on your work history. Is there somewhere you could see the need for an SOP? What? Where? Why?

Resources and References

1. Pharmacy Compounding (795) In: *United States Pharmacopeia 25/National Formulary* 20. Rockville, MD: United States Pharmacopeial Convention, 2001.
2. Pharmaceutical Compounding—Sterile Preparations In: *United States Pharmacopeia 27/National Formulary* 22. Rockville, MD: United States Pharmacopeial Convention, 2003.

CHAPTER 5

Capsules, Tablets, and Powders

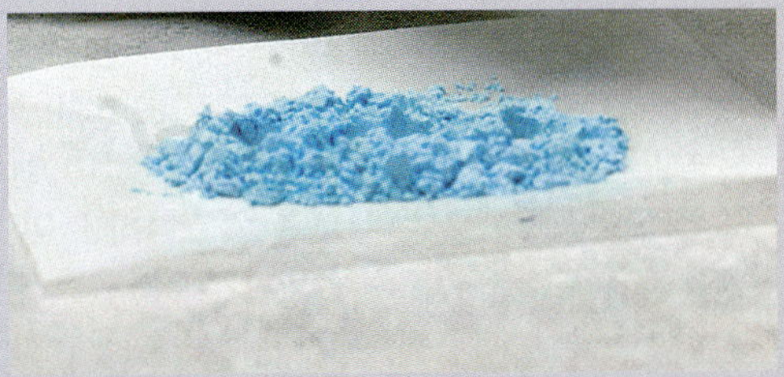

Learning Objectives

After completing this chapter, you should be able to:

- Distinguish the different types of capsules, tablets, and powders.
- List the ingredients and composition properties required to prepare capsules, tablets, and powders.
- Explain the procedures and techniques used to prepare capsules, tablets, and powders.
- Describe how to perform quality control testing of capsules, tablets, and powders.
- Select appropriate packaging for the compounded capsules, tablets, and powders.
- List the labeling requirements for capsules, tablets, and powders.
- Evaluate the stability of capsules, tablets, and powders.

INTRODUCTION

Capsules, tablets, and powders are among the most common dosage forms of medication. With these dosage forms, the compounding pharmacy can customize medications to meet individual patient requirements while still providing an easy and convenient route of administration.

Types and Definitions

The first dosage form to be discussed will be capsules.

CAPSULES

A **capsule** is a solid dosage form in which the active ingredient and any necessary excipients are enclosed in either a soft or a hard soluble gelatin shell that will dissolve in the stomach, releasing the medication. The contents of a capsule may be semisolid, powder, or liquid. They are usually swallowed whole, but in some instances may be opened and the contents mixed with food or liquid. Capsules can also be administered rectally or vaginally to deliver an exact prescribed dose, depending on the disease state and the desired results of the prescriber. Capsules are a versatile dosage form in that they can be formulated for an immediate release or a delayed release, they may contain

capsule
a solid dosage form in which the active ingredient and any necessary excipients are enclosed in either a soft or hard soluble gelatin shell

more than one active ingredient, and they offer dosing flexibility for the prescriber. Some of the benefits of capsules include pharmaceutical elegance, convenience, ease of administration, and relative taste concealment. Capsules are tasteless, easy to swallow, and offer an alternative to extremely bitter, unpleasant-tasting, or offensive-smelling drugs commercially available only in liquid form.

Capsules can be easily compounded extemporaneously on the basis of the individual need of a patient. Not only can a capsule be formulated to contain the exact dose of medication needed according to a patient's weight or specific disease protocol, but they can also be formulated to contain several medications in a single dose. This makes dosing easier for the patient or caregiver, and it enhances compliancy as well. In addition, having several medications compounded into one prescription will often be more cost effective.

For certain people who may be sensitive or allergic to certain excipients, such as preservatives, dyes, or lactose, the compounded capsule offers a solution that allows the patient to get the needed medication, while leaving out the agent that could be problematic. For example, a patient who is sensitive to certain preservatives or dyes could have a capsule compounded containing the active ingredient only. Of course, stability of the chemical must be studied beforehand to make sure the drug is stable in a preservative-free environment.

Capsules are also extemporaneously compounded when a manufacturer discontinues a drug because of low sales or declining use. There are some individuals who may still benefit from the active ingredient for its intended use or for another "off label" use. In other cases, drugs that have been pulled from the human market by the Food and Drug Administration are often still necessary for the treatment of specific disorders in animals.

For the patient who cannot swallow tablets, but can ingest a capsule, the compounding pharmacy is invaluable. Similar is the situation where a needed dose is available only in an offensive-tasting liquid. A capsule can be formulated that offers the prescriber and the patient a tasteless and convenient option to getting the necessary medication. A capsule may also be compounded when a tablet is available only in a certain dose range that is not applicable to the patient's disease state or is inappropriate for his weight. Rather than cut the tablet and risk getting a **sub-therapeutic** or **super-therapeutic** dose, or having the patient take more than one tablet in order to achieve the desired dose, a capsule may be compounded to the exact required dose.

sub-therapeutic
below the desired beneficial result

super-therapeutic
above the desired beneficial result

TABLETS

tablet
solid dosage form that may be administered orally, sublingually, vaginally, or as an implant or pellet under the skin

Tablets are a solid dosage form that may be administered orally, sublingually, vaginally, or as an implant or pellet under the skin. The *compressed tablet* is probably the most prescribed dosage form. This is because it is convenient, portable, stable, and for the most part easy to administer. The single disadvantage to commercially made tablets is that they are available only in fixed dosage strengths and combinations. The compounding pharmacy has always had the ability to compound molded tablets; and now, with the advent of pellet presses and single punch tablet presses, compressed tablets can be prepared according to the requirements of specific patients.

There are several different forms of tablets that can be compounded. These include *sublingual tablets*, which are placed under the tongue; *tablet triturates*, which dissolve in body fluids; *buccal tablets*, which are placed in the cheek pouch to dissolve; compressed tablets, which are designed to be swallowed whole; rapid-dissolving tablets, which dissolve instantly when placed in the oral cavity; effervescent tablets, which are submersed in a liquid to dissolve and then are consumed by the patient; and implants or pellets, which are imbedded in the body subcutaneously. One other tablet form is for hypodermic administration. This form is prepared aseptically and mixed with a *diluent* prior to injection.

Tablet triturates, sublingual tablets, buccal tablets, and rapid-dissolve tablets are all considered molded tablets. These types of tablets are prepared in a mold of appropriate size for the intended dosage form and use. The typical die plate cavity size ranges from 60 mg to 100 mg, which limits the size of tablet that can be made. All are prepared similarly, with the use of calibrated molds that are either plastic or metal.

POWDERS

Powders are a solid dosage form made from a thoroughly blended mixture of one or more active ingredients and excipients. Powders, as a pharmaceutical dosage form, may be used either internally or externally. Powders for reconstitution, such as those used to prepare antibiotics, oral powders, and powders administered with an insufflator into a body cavity, are all examples of internally used powders. External powders include those used for dusting a compromised area of skin with medicinal products, such as an antifungal.

powders
a solid dosage form made from blended mixture of active ingredients and excipients

Although the use of powders has declined, there is still the occasional need for a powder to be prescribed. Both pediatric and geriatric patients who either are unable to swallow or have extreme difficulty swallowing tablets or capsules can benefit from having their medication in powder form. The caregiver or the patient can simply mix the medicinal powder with food or liquid for ingestion. A powder dosage form may also be prepared if a drug is too bulky to prepare in capsule or tablet form.

Powders that are inhaled through the nostril to treat headaches have been around for many years and are still commercially available today. Variations on these products may be compounded, offering a more therapeutic benefit in treating the migraine sufferer. Occasionally, a prescriber will want to treat a disease state with a unique approach such as **insufflation** of powder into the ear canal or nasal passage. An example of this type of treatment is the use of an antibacterial, such as sulfanilamide, that is puffed into the ear canal by using an insufflator. Premeasured powder packets are prepared and usually dispensed with an insufflator, or the medication may be dispensed directly inside the insufflator. The medication may be used by the patient, or the physician may wish to administer the drug in his office. Dermatologists

insufflation
to blow onto or in

may order powder preparations for their patients to treat such conditions as athlete's foot. In this case, an antifungal such as miconazole may be mixed with a dusting powder such as corn starch or talc, which will have a drying effect on the skin.

Powder dosage forms are not uncommon in veterinary medicine. For the equine patient, a bitter drug such as pergolide can be mixed with dextrose or sucrose powder, offering the owner a convenient and easy alternative to trying to pill the horse or administer a liquid. The bulk powder is usually prepared so that the desired dose is contained in 5 grams of the appropriate sugar. A scoop that will measure 5 grams is dispensed with the powder. The owner then can simply sprinkle the medicated powder on the animal's food. It is important in the dispensing process to go over the instructions for measuring the exact dose with the owner or caregiver. If the required dose is contained in one level scoop of the measuring device, then it should be *communicated* that the excess powder in the scoop must be scraped off with a straight edge such as the back of a knife. This will ensure that the patient receives the exact prescribed dose of the medication.

Composition and Ingredients

The gelatin shell used in capsules is made of two parts. The base is the longer end and fits into the shorter end, which is referred to as the cap. The cap is designed to fit over the base and then snap or lock into place with added pressure (Figure 5-1).

opaque
not reflecting light; dark

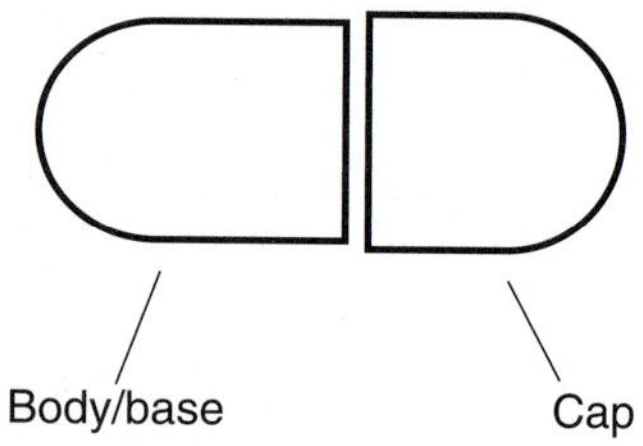

Figure 5-1 Components of a capsule

Capsules are oval in shape and available in eight different sizes for human use. These sizes are #5, #4, #3, #2, #1, #0, #00, and #000, with the smallest being a #5 and the largest a #000. The numbers used to designate size have no bearing on the volume that may be contained within. The capacity of a capsule is dependent on the density and physical characteristics of the powders used in the formula (Figure 5-2).

There are additional capsule sizes available for veterinary compounding. These are #10, #11, and #12. The relative capacities for these sizes are 1 ounce, $\frac{1}{2}$ ounce, and $\frac{1}{4}$ ounce, respectively. The #5 and #4 capsules are also frequently used when formulating capsules for smaller animal patients.

Empty capsules are available as clear, opaque, and colored. **Opaque** capsules are used when a fixed oil is necessary either to dissolve or suspend the

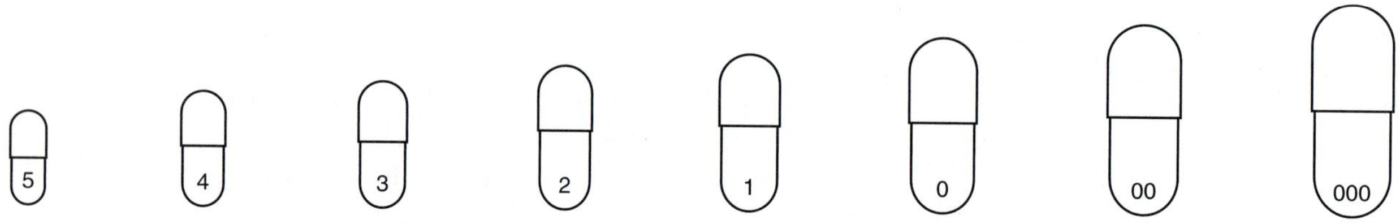

Figure 5-2 Capsule size chart

drug or because the chemical is stable only in a fixed-oil environment. Opaque or colored capsules may also be used if a drug is light sensitive, such as cyclosporine. This is an added assurance, even though most capsules are dispensed in an amber vial. The reason for using opaque capsules is pharmaceutical elegance. Air will inevitably be trapped in the cap, and a bubble will form in the oil. Using opaque capsules will prevent the consumer from seeing the bubble. Colored capsules are used to designate different medications or different strengths of the same medication. A coloring agent may be added to the powders to be encapsulated in a clear shell, producing a colored capsule. This is necessary when a patient is receiving more than one compounded capsule or, again, to designate strength when more than one strength of a particular drug is routinely compounded in the pharmacy. In addition, an approved coloring agent is sometimes added to the formula to ensure that the active ingredient is uniformly dispersed throughout the mixture. This is useful especially when the amount of drug being incorporated is very small when compared with the total amount of excipients needed. For example, a formula calls for 23 mg of levothyroxine to be mixed with 10 mg of powdered colorant and 14.5 g of spray dried lactose to produce a quantity of powder needed to fill 100 #4 capsules, so that each of the finished capsules will contain 0.23 mg of levothyroxine. Because of the added color, the final mixture can be examined for uniform dispersion.

The relationship between the active ingredient and the necessary excipients will vary with each compounded capsule prescription. The key factor that must be taken into consideration is the physical property of each powder used in the formula. Granular and crystalline powders do not pack well when the capsule is filled by hand. However, both of these types of powders flow well and readily fall into the empty body of the capsule when a capsule machine is used. The inverse is true when working with soft, fluffy powders. These types of powders will pack easily into capsules when hand filled, but require more manipulation or possibly an additive, such as magnesium stearate or sodium lauryl sulfate, to enhance manageability of the chemical when a capsule machine is used. The additive may either improve the chemical's ability to flow or reduce static electricity in the chemical, making it easier to work with. The nature of the chemical will determine the best method for encapsulation as well as which additives might be most beneficial when compounding capsules with a drug that is otherwise difficult to manipulate.

Tablets are generally prepared by using the active ingredient along with excipients such as lactose, sucrose, dextrose, manitol, or a combination of sugars that form an appropriate base. Drugs that react chemically with sugars will require special bases such as precipitated calcium carbonate, precipitated calcium phosphate, or kaolin. Whichever base is used, it must be soluble and should not degrade during preparation.

Some bulk chemicals are used as powder dose in their pure state. One example of this is the use of sucralfate in equine patients; another is tylosin tartrate, an antibiotic used to treat felines and canines. It is also common for farm animals to receive **prophylactic** medications from powders mixed in their drinking supply.

prophylactic
preventive measure or medication

Preparation and Compounding Techniques

The preparation and compounding techniques vary depending upon whether a capsule, tablet or powder is involved.

CAPSULES

In many instances it will be necessary to calculate the capacity of the capsule being compounded. This can be done by filling the capsule completely with the active ingredient and recording the amount. Next, fill an empty capsule of the same size with the appropriate excipient and record this amount. The amount needed to deliver an exact dose of the active ingredient is then divided by the total amount of active ingredient the capsule will hold. This figure is expressed as a percentage representing the portion of needed active ingredient to be contained in the capsule. This figure is then subtracted from 100 percent. Finally, the total amount of excipient is multiplied by the remaining difference in the percentage, giving the amount of filler needed to accurately bring the capsule to volume.

Example:

The total amount of Hydroxyzine HCl a #4 capsule will hold is 100 mg.
The prescription is written for 37.5 mg of Hydroxyzine HCl.
37.5 mg is divided by 100 mg, giving a percentage of 37.5.
The total amount of spray dried lactose that a #4 will hold is 145 mg.
145 mg is multiplied by the difference in the percentage, which is 62.5 percent.
$0.145 \text{ gm} \times 62.5\% = 0.090 \text{ gm}$ per capsule
Each capsule will contain 37.5 mg of Hydroxyzine and 90 mg of spray dried lactose.
These numbers are then multiplied by the total number of capsules needed to fill the prescription.

To save time when compounding capsules, it may be helpful to design a chart listing the capacities of frequently used chemicals and excipients for the different capsule sizes. There are various printed charts available for common excipients, such as Table 5-1.

TABLE 5-1 Example Capsule Capacity Chart

Capsule Size	Lactose	Avicel PH-105	Starch	Methocel E4M	Kaolin	Methocel K100 m	Calcium CO3
#4	190 mg	110 mg	180 mg	100 mg	165 mg	100 mg	220 mg
#3	225 mg	130 mg	205 mg	150 mg	250 mg	150 mg	275 mg
#2	300 mg	160 mg	285 mg	188 mg	375 mg	185 mg	350 mg
#1	400 mg	230 mg	375 mg	250 mg	540 mg	250 mg	460 mg
#0	550 mg	320 mg	510 mg	350 mg	600 mg	350 mg	640 mg
#00	775 mg	450 mg	700 mg	475 mg	765 mg	475 mg	925 mg
#000	1260 mg	725 mg	1180 mg	620 mg	1700 mg	620 mg	1450 mg

The active ingredients and excipients needed to form the capsule may be encapsulated by hand or by using a capsule machine. Which method is best will be determined by several different factors. When preparing a prescription for a relatively low number of doses where a bulky powder is being used, it is generally easier and quicker to fill the capsules by hand. If preparing a larger number of capsules, such as 100, it will usually be more efficient for the preparer to use a capsule machine. Physicochemical considerations that should be taken into account are the **density** of the powder(s), the ease in which they flow, static electricity, and the total amount of powder to be encapsulated.

density
the amount of darkness or light in an area of a scan that reflects the compactness and density of tissue

All ingredients should be compared with those listed on the formula worksheet. Calculations for the total amounts needed are done twice to ensure accuracy and confirmed by the pharmacist. Each ingredient is then carefully weighed, and the amount is confirmed by the pharmacist. (As individual state laws allow, the weights may be checked by another pharmacy technician.)

WORKPLACE WISDOM

When preparing any compounded prescription, the ingredients should be checked at least three times throughout the compounding procedure.

Powder ingredients to be encapsulated should be comminuted to reduce particle size. This may be done by using a mortar and pestle, by passing the powders through a size 100 sieve, or by using a powder blender. After the particle size has been reduced, the ingredients should be mixed together, using the principle of geometric dilution. This is to start with the ingredient of the smallest amount and double the portion by adding the additional ingredients in order of quantity. Each addition should result in a "doubled" amount until all the ingredients are mixed in. This process ensures even distribution of the active ingredient throughout the final mixture.

When all the ingredients have been combined, the capsules are ready to be filled and weighed. First, however, the scale must be prepared. This is done by placing an empty capsule, both cap and bottom, onto a piece of weighing paper on the scale. The scale is then tared, or zeroed out. The weights that will now be displayed on the scale will be for the contents of the capsule only, and not the shell or weigh paper.

Hand Filling

When filling a capsule by hand, the powder is poured out onto a clean sheet of paper on a hard surface such as a countertop. It is then packed by using the flat side of a spatula or by folding the piece of paper over the powder and gently pressing a flat hand down onto the powder. Next, the long end of the capsule is pushed into the powder. It is sometimes helpful to rotate the capsule body a quarter of a turn as it comes in contact with the surface below. This process is repeated until the capsule contains the exact amount of the powder needed to accurately deliver the prescribed dose. The capsules are weighed individually as they are being filled. Each weighing will determine whether more powder is needed or if some of the powder inside the capsule should be removed. An error rate of 10 percent or less is acceptable (Figure 5-3 A-G).

Machine Filling

When using a capsule machine, a powder dam is clamped into place on the top work surface to prevent any powder from falling over the edges. The powder mixture is then poured over the exposed capsule bases, which have been loaded into the machine. The powder is then moved around the surface by gently shaking or

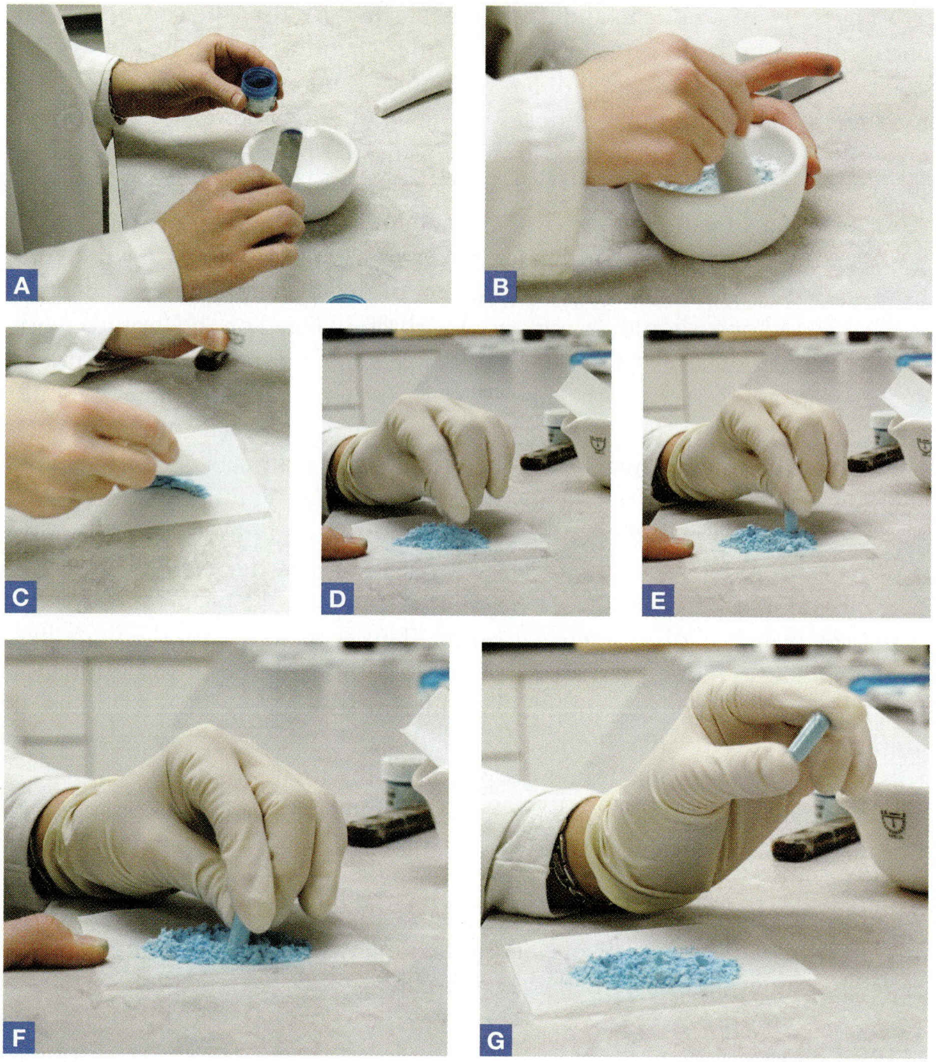

Figure 5-3 Filling a capsule by hand

rocking the machine back and forth or by using a powder scraper to push the powder over the openings holding the capsule bases. As the powder uniformly drops into the bases, the machine can be gently tapped on the countertop so the powder will drop. A tamping device is then used to pack the powder down into the body of the capsule. The tamper is available in a variety of sizes. A five-pronged tamper is most efficient, especially for bulky powders. This process is repeated until the capsules are evenly filled and all the powder has been distributed. Next, the filled bases should be examined to make sure all the capsules are evenly filled. Finally, the caps are put on and then locked into place (Figure 5-4 A-M).

A sample weighing of the finished capsules should be performed. This is done by individually weighing 10 of the capsules to make sure they are within 10 percent of the required weight. Ten of the capsules should also be weighed as a group and an average weight calculated. Again, this figure should be within 10 percent of the needed weight. These sample weights should be recorded on the formula worksheet.

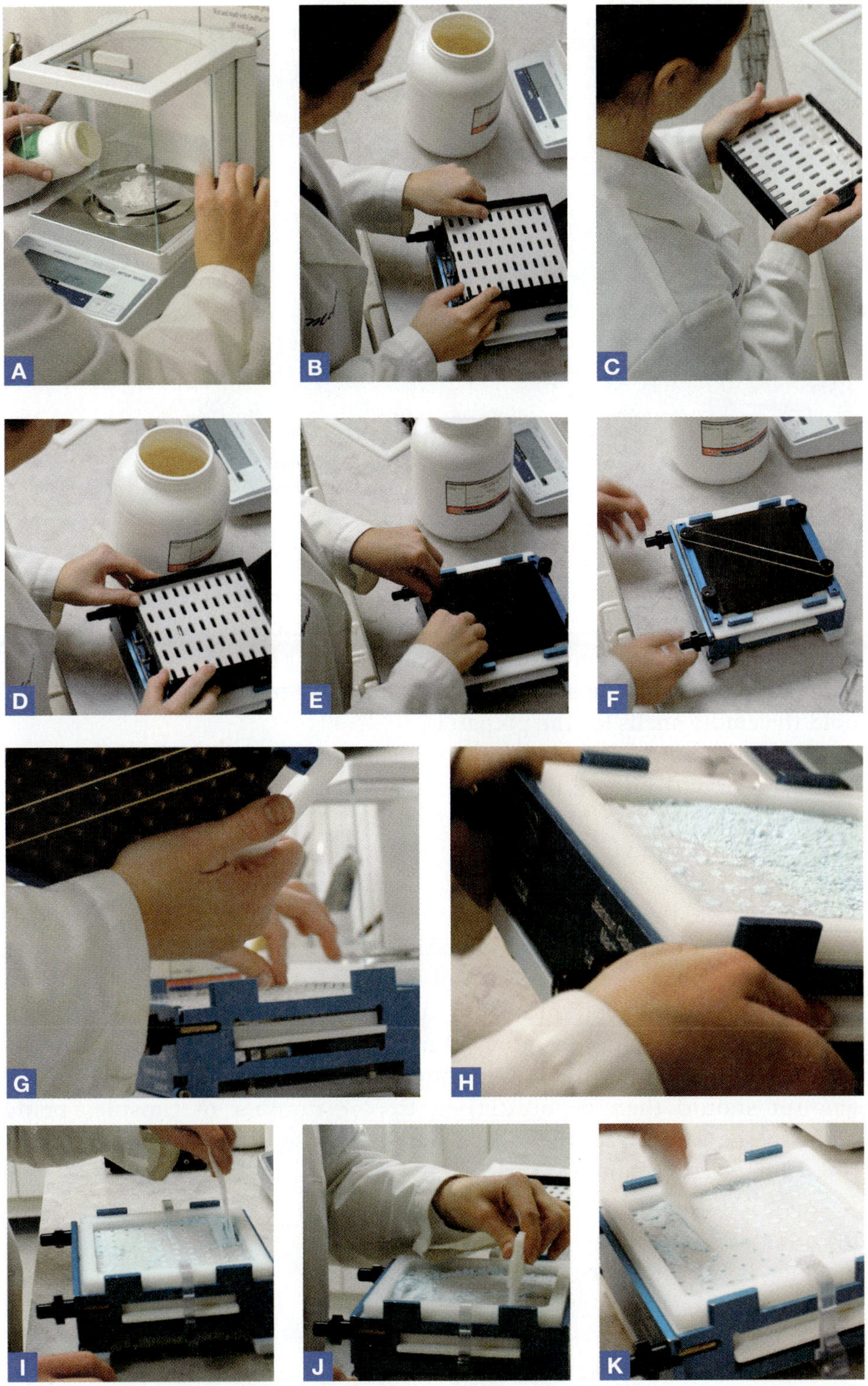

Figure 5-4 Using a capsule machine

Figure 5-4 Using a capsule machine (*continued*)

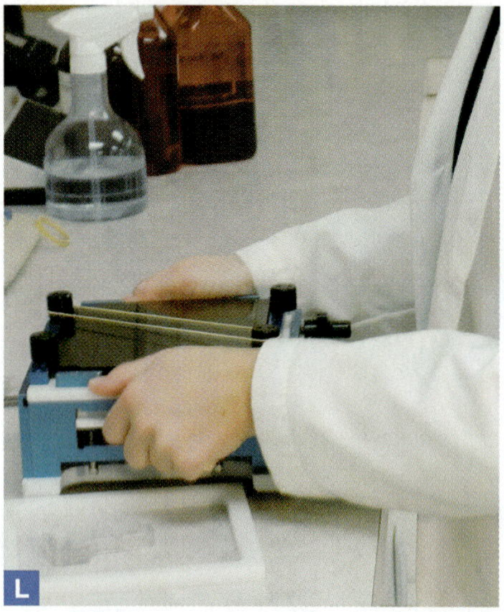

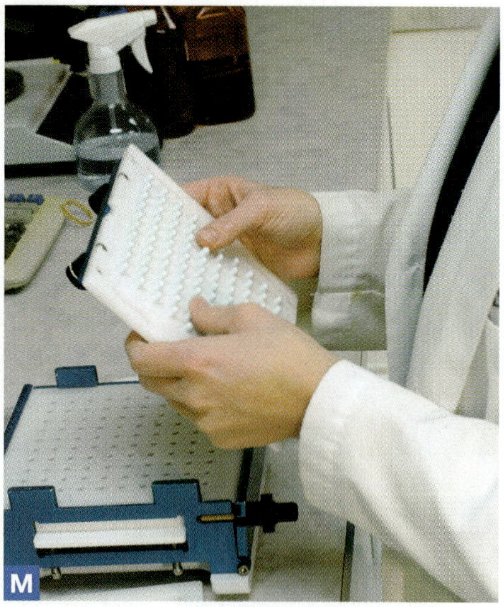

Oil Filled Capsules

Certain drugs are stable only in a fixed-oil environment. Although an oral liquid may be prepared, it is also possible to prepare capsules filled with oil. The process is tedious and requires a steady hand. The capsules may be filled by hand, but using a capsule machine can make the task easier since it will hold the empty shells for the preparer.

WORKPLACE WISDOM

When oil filled capsules are prepared, the total amount should always be calculated for 10 percent more than is needed. This will allow for partial loss due to residue left behind in the mortar as well as the syringe, and possible overflow or spillage when the capsules are filled.

First, the empty capsules must be calibrated. To do this, fill a 10ml oral syringe with the oil base used in the formula. Carefully fill 10 capsules drop wise. The machine should be tapped on a hard surface to allow any air that may be trapped at the bottom of the capsule base to escape. When all 10 capsules are completely full, the meniscus should be visible just below the top of each capsule. (Care must be taken so that the capsules are not overfilled, creating a crowning effect of the oil and causing leaking of the finished product.) After the 10 capsules are properly filled, note the amount of oil remaining in the oral syringe. Subtract the difference from the original 10 ml. Divide this amount by 10 to determine the amount of oil contained in each capsule. The resulting amount should then be multiplied by the number of capsules being made in the formula. This will be the figure used for bringing the mixture to its final volume (Figure 5-5 A-L).

Figure 5-5 Filling capsules with oil

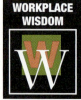

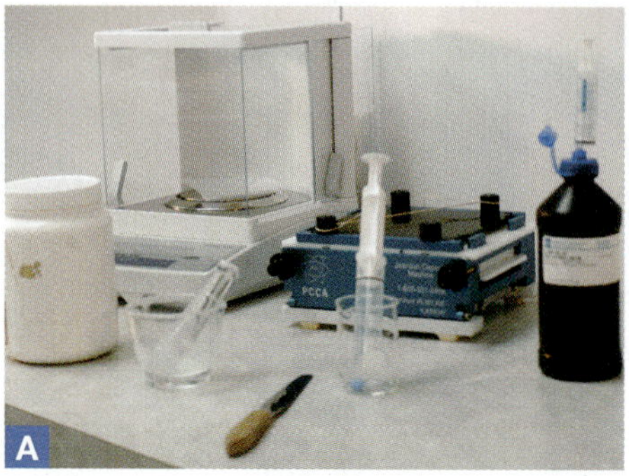

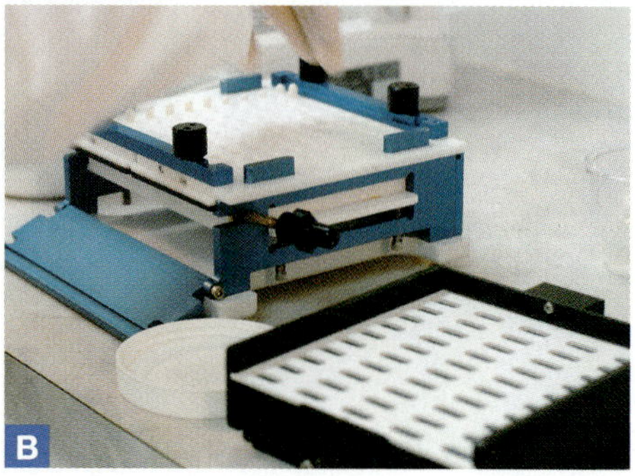

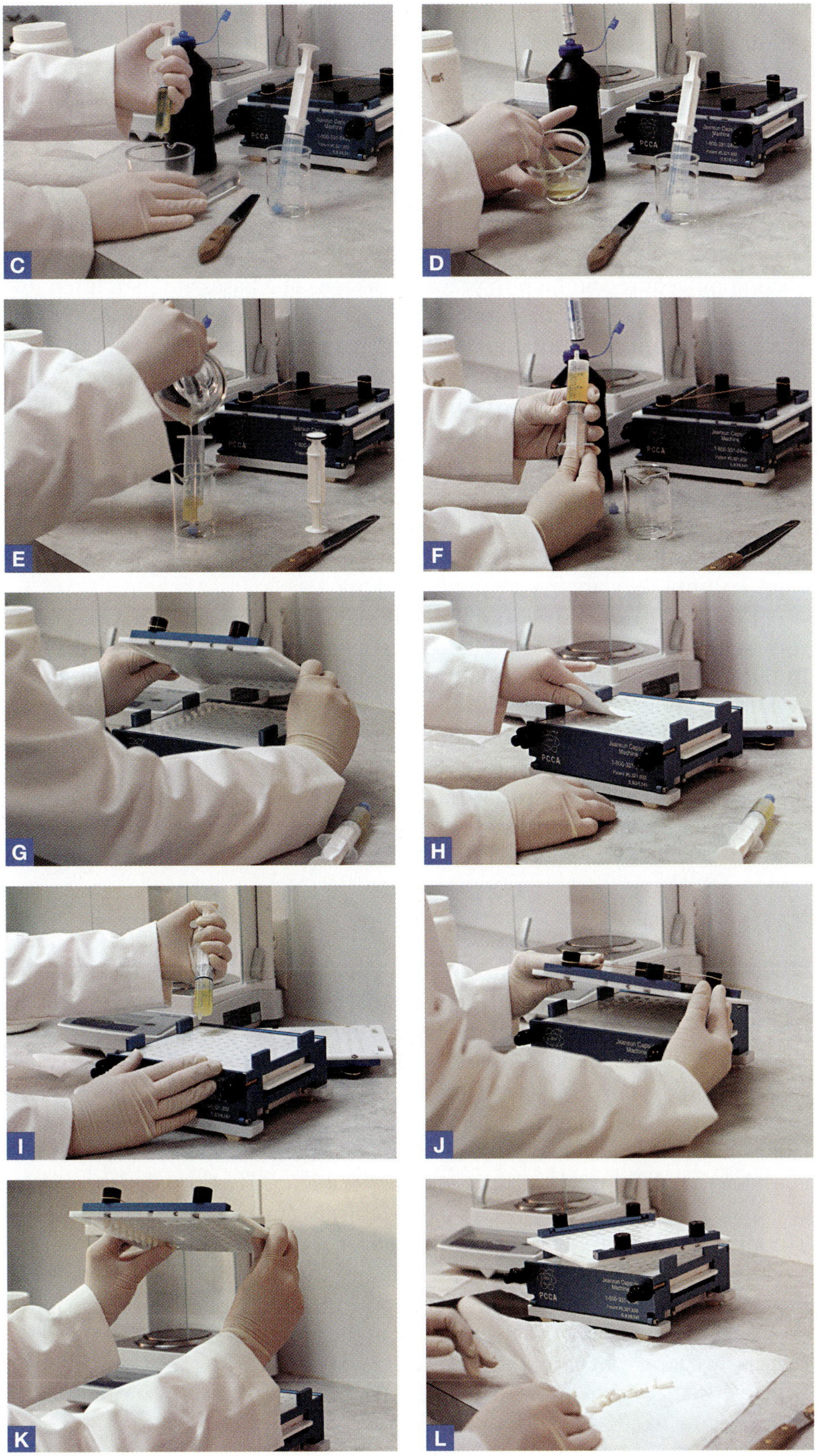

Figure 5-5 Filling capsules with oil (*continued*)

When incorporating the active ingredient, the principle of geometric dilution, as discussed earlier, is applied. While some drugs will dissolve in oil, other heavier drugs will displace the oil. This factor must be taken into consideration when determining the amounts of active ingredient(s) and any other excipients needed in the formula.

When all the ingredients have been properly mixed, the capsules may then be filled by following the preceding method. To prepare the caps for assembly, it is helpful to take a cloth dampened with distilled water and wipe the underneath side of the top plate holding the caps. This will aid in the caps locking procedure and help to prevent leakage. The bases are then lifted into the caps. Next, the top plate holding the capsules is lifted out of the capsule machine without inverting the plate. The bases are then locked into place by gently pressing on each one from underneath the plate holding them. Because of the air trapped in the cap, the capsules may pop back down, causing them not to lock. Repeating the process of locking the capsules may be necessary until they are securely joined (Figure 5-6 A-I).

When all the capsules are sufficiently locked, they can be removed from the plate. They should be placed on an absorbent towel and the excess oil removed. This is done by folding the cloth over them and gently rolling the capsules until they are free of any oil residue.

If the practitioner desires a long-acting medication to be compounded, this can be accomplished by incorporating a methylcellulose type product into the mixture. There are different products as well as different grades of cellulose products. The type of product or grade to be used will be determined by the drug being compounded. Usually, this information will be supplied on published formulas or recipes. If there is no existing formula for a particular drug, research must be done to avoid using an incorrect product, which may react with the chemical or result in a drug being released too quickly or too slowly.

TABLETS

Calibrating the mold is done prior to compounding a specific formula, since each base will have a different capacity. This is done by preparing a sample batch of the base used in the formula. Ten of the cavities in the mold are filled to capacity, left to set, and then carefully removed and weighed. The entire sample batch is weighed and then divided by the number of tablets in the sample. This gives the weight for each individual tablet. This figure is used when performing the calculations in the formula. The physical properties of the active ingredient must be considered. **Solubility** of the drug and the total amount of powder(s) to be incorporated will determine whether or not a displacement factor must be used. If a formula does not give the displacement factor, this can be calculated by wetting a portion of the active ingredient and filling 10 cavities. After they dry, they can be removed and weighed. A percentage is then figured by dividing the required dose by the total amount of active ingredient the mold will hold. This will tell the preparer what percentage of the filled cavity will be made up of active ingredient, with the balance being for the base. It is advisable to calculate the formula for 10 percent extra, to allow for loss during preparation of the tablets.

solubility
the degree of being able to dissolve into

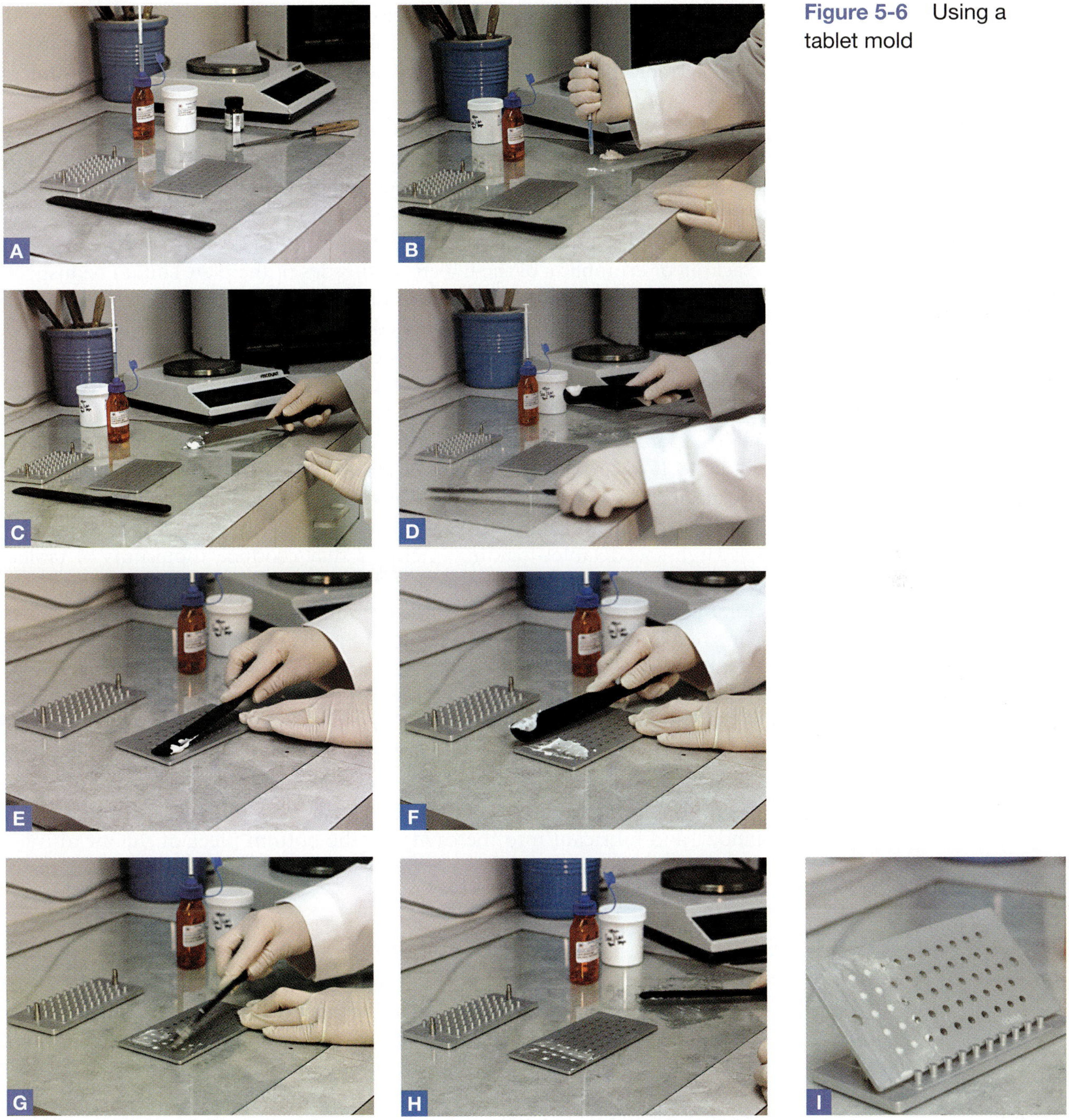

Figure 5-6 Using a tablet mold

The active ingredient is triturated with the tablet base in geometric proportion. When the powders are thoroughly combined, the mixture is then dampened to the consistency of play dough so that it is pliable and will adhere to the mold. This is usually done with a mixture of ethanol and distilled or preserved water (typically 50 to 80 percent alcohol). Proper consistency is important. If the mixture is too wet, the sugars in the base will dissolve. If it is too dry, it will crack or crumble before the tablets can be properly formed. This is a learned skill that will develop with experience.

The mold plate should be placed on a glass surface such as an ointment tile. The wetted mixture is then forced into the holes of the top plate by using a hard rubber spatula and applying sufficient pressure to adequately pack each cavity. (A stainless steel spatula is not recommended as it can scratch the surface of the mold plate.) The tops are smoothed with the flat edge of a spatula, and any gross excess is removed. The preparer must work quickly and efficiently to fill the holes of the mold before the mixture dries in order to prevent cracking or crumbling of the tablets. Both sides of the plate should be inspected for any obvious unfilled space within the cavities. While the tablets are still somewhat moist, the top plate is aligned over the bottom plate, which has pegs on it. The top plate is then gently pressed down, allowing the pegs to push the tablets out of the holes, and is left to rest on the tops of the pegs to dry. When the tablets are completely dry, they are carefully removed and transferred to a piece of porous material such as cheese cloth, which will allow for nonrestricted air to flow around the tablets to ensure thorough drying. They are then packaged in air-tight containers, labeled with the proper auxiliary label concerning storage, and are ready to be dispensed to the patient.

WORKPLACE WISDOM

Hint: Unit dose packaging, if possible, will prevent breakage from the fragile tablets bumping into each other or the inside of the vial during transportation.

High-speed tablet-making machines that produce thousands of tablets per batch are commonly used in the pharmaceutical industry. A small variation on these machines, called a single-punch tablet press, is available to prepare extemporaneously compounded tablets at the pharmacy level. Compressed tablets in the past were made rarely and only in unique situations. As technology has evolved, more and more pharmacies that compound are offering this dosage form.

The different types of tablets made by using a tablet press are chewable tablets, effervescent tablets, and compressed tablets. The tablets are made by placing a combined mixture of active ingredient, a diluent, a disintegrant, a binder, and lubricant into the cavity on the bottom piece of the metal tube. The handle on the tablet press is depressed and released. The powders are compressed, thus producing the tablet.

POWDERS

trituration
the process of reducing the particle size of a substance by grinding it (typically with a mortar and pestle)

The particle size of the active ingredient and any excipients must be reduced so that all the particles of each ingredient are of the same size. Since particles of a larger size will settle at a faster rate, there is a risk that the active ingredient will separate out of the mixture. To ensure that the particles are equal in size, each powder should be passed through a size 100 mesh sieve, or **triturated** by using a Wedgwood, glass, or ceramic mortar and pestle, or by using an electric powder blender. Which method is used will depend on the physical characteristics of the ingredients in the preparation. For example, potent drugs or drugs with a narrow therapeutic index should be comminuted in a nonporous mortar, such as glass, so that no drug will be lost in the pores or the mortar, resulting in a subtherapeutic dose for the patient or causing cross contamination with the next product prepared in that mortar. For most other situations, Wedgwood or porcelain mortars and pestles are appropriate when working with powders.

When mixing powders to prepare a powder dosage form, it is absolutely critical that the principle of geometric dilution be applied. This is to start with the ingredient of smallest quantity and add the remaining ingredients in order of quantity by "doubling" the original amount until all the ingredients have been thoroughly mixed together. Mixing can be accomplished by using a mortar and pestle, a bottle, a plastic bag sealed with air inside, a sieve, or a sifter.

When working with extremely light and fluffy powders, the preparer may choose to wear a dust mask and goggles to prevent inhaling the fine particles that may escape into the air. An additive such as magnesium stearate (less than one percent) will act as a lubricant and thus enhance the flow characteristics of such fluffy powders. Likewise, using sodium lauryl sulfate (up to one percent) will reduce static electricity in powders that tend to "fly away" or are difficult to work with.

Some powders may become sticky with manipulation. This can be avoided by mixing in a bulky powder adsorbent such as light magnesium oxide or magnesium carbonate. These powders should be triturated very lightly on a pill tile, using a spatula to mix rather than a mortar and pestle.

Certain chemicals may react or interact with certain excipients. It is important to research such things before compounding any prescription. For example, fluoxetine powder is not stable when compounded with lactose. A fluoxetine capsule must be compounded with avicel or no filler at all.

Quality Control

As with any compounded formula, quality control procedures should be performed on the final product. Capsules, tablets, and powders should be inspected for appearance, proper weight, and signs of disintegration. A sample weighing of individual doses should be performed and an average weight recorded. A weight on the total sample divided by the number of doses in the sample should be performed and recorded as well.

Packaging

Capsules and tablets should be packaged in light-resistant vials. Hygroscopic and deliquescent powders will absorb moisture from the air to the extent that they will become moist or even liquefy. The powders should be completely dry in order to be presentable to the patient. To ensure that the product remains dry and acceptable, it should be dispensed in an air-tight container with a desiccant. Powders dispensed in individual doses may be packaged in neatly folded, secure powder papers.

Labeling

The following information should be included on all compounding labels: generic or chemical name of the active ingredient(s), strength and/or quantity, an assigned pharmacy lot number, beyond-use or expiration date, storage requirements, and instructions for use.

Stability

If no information is available, beyond-use dates are assigned as described in the section "Stability Criteria and Beyond-Use Dating" in the general test chapter "Pharmaceutical Compounding Nonsterile Preparations ⟨795⟩." Extended beyond-use dates may be used if supported by appropriate literature sources such as published studies in journals, or by direct testing evidence.

Patient Counseling

The patient or caregiver should be asked if he or she would like counseling about the compound from the pharmacist. Instructions for use, including how often the drug is taken, duration of therapy, and the importance completing the entire therapy as well as any pertinent storage requirements, should be expressed.

SUMMARY

While capsules, tablets, and powders are by far the most common dosage forms of medication, there are still numerous opportunities for a compounding pharmacy to meet the needs of an individual patient through a custom compound. Each dosage form requires special equipment and a learned technique to provide a safe, efficacious, and pharmaceutically elegant compound.

PROFILES OF PRACTICE

Sample Formula: Placebo Capsules

for training purposes only—using a size 0 capsule

Lactose NF Hydrous	54 g
Silica Gel Micronized	0.2 g
Powdered Food Color	0.1 g

1. Accurately measure each ingredient.
2. Using geometric dilution, mix powders together.
3. Sift through a mesh sieve into a weight boat or directly onto the capsule machine.
4. Fill capsules according to directions for the capsule machine.
5. Place in container and label.

Makes 100 "0-size" capsules.

Sample Formula: Ibuprofen 200 mg Tablets

for training purposes only

Ibuprofen	20 g
Caffeine	10 g
Avicel PH 101	14 g
Stearic acid	200 mg

1. Accurately measure each ingredient.
2. Using geometric dilution, mix the powders, starting with the ibuprofen and caffeine, then avicel, and finally the stearic acid.
3. Weigh 442 mg of the mixture, place it in the tablet press, and prepare the tablets.
4. Place in container and label.

Sample Formula: Bulk Oral Powder

for training purposes only for use as an electrolyte and rehydration solution

Dextrose	25 g
Sodium Chloride	2.5 g
Potassium Citrate	4.5 g

1. Accurately measure each ingredient.
2. Mix together all ingredients.
3. Place in container and label to dilute with 1 L of liquid for drinking.

CHAPTER TERMS

capsule
a solid dosage form in which the active ingredient and any necessary excipients are enclosed in either a soft or hard soluble gelatin shell

density
the amount of darkness or light in an area of a scan that reflects the compactness and density of tissue

insufflation
to blow onto or in

opaque
not reflecting light; dark

powder
a solid dosage form made from blended mixture of active ingredients and excipients

prophylactic
preventive measure or medication

solubility
the degree of being able to dissolve into

sub-therapeutic
below the desired beneficial result

super-therapeutic
above the desired beneficial result

tablet
solid dosage form that may be administered orally, sublingually, vaginally, or as an implant or pellet under the skin

trituration
the process of reducing the particle size of a substance by grinding it (typically with a mortar and pestle)

CHAPTER 5

CHAPTER REVIEW QUESTIONS

1. A solid dosage form in which the active ingredient and any necessary excipients are enclosed in either a soft or hard soluble gelatin shell that will dissolve in the stomach releasing the medication is called
   a. a troche
   b. a capsule
   c. a suppository
   d. a lozenge

2. A solid dosage form that may be administered orally, sublingually, vaginally, or as an implant or pellet under the skin is known as
   a. a tablet
   b. a capsule
   c. a troche
   d. a suppository

3. Which of the following is a disadvantage for tablet form?
   a. tablets are too hard
   b. cannot put too many milligrams in a tablet
   c. dosing is set amount
   d. cannot use certain fillers

4. What can be added to help avoid some sticky powders with manipulation?
   a. fixed oil ingredients
   b. light magnesium oxide
   c. magnesium carbonate
   d. both b and c

5. The typical die plate cavity size for tablet molds ranges from
   a. 5 mg to 100 mg
   b. 10 mg to 100 mg
   c. 60 mg to 100 mg
   d. 50 mg to 100 mg

6. True or false: While compounding a prescription, it is advised to check the prescription three times.
   a. true
   b. false

7. True or false: The process of blowing a fine powder into the ear canal or nasal passage is known as mitigation.
   a. true
   b. false

8. How many different sizes of capsule forms are available?

9. Describe where each of the following are placed:
   a. sublingual tablets
   b. tablet triturates
   c. buccal tablets

10. **Critical Thinking** When and why should opaque capsules be used in compounding?

Resources and References

1. Allen, Loyd V. Jr., Ph.D. *The Art, Science, and Technology of Pharmaceutical Compounding*. Washington, DC: American Pharmaceutical Association, 1998.
2. *Remington's Pharmaceutical Sciences*, 15th Edition. Easton, PA: Mack Publishing Co. 1975.
3. Allen, Loyd V. Jr., Ph.D. *Secundum Artem: Compounding Suppositories, Part I*. Vol. 3, No. 3, Minneapolis, MN.
4. Allen, Loyd V. Jr., Ph.D. *Secundum Artem: Compounding Suppositories, Part II*. Vol. 3, No. 4, Minneapolis, MN.
5. Shrewsbury, Robert, *Applied Pharmaceutics in Contemporary Compounding*. Morton Publishing, 2001.

CHAPTER 6

Lozenges, Troches, Sticks, and Suppositories

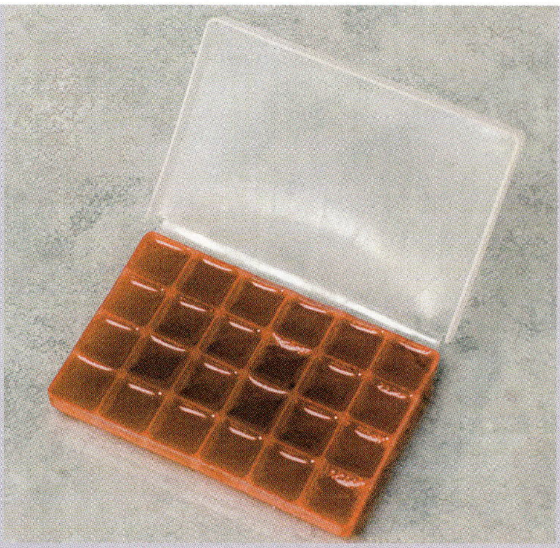

Learning Objectives

After completing this chapter, you should be able to:

- Distinguish the different types of lozenges, troches, sticks, and suppositories.
- List the ingredients and composition properties required to prepare lozenges, troches, sticks, and suppositories.
- Explain the procedures and techniques used to prepare lozenges, troches, sticks, and suppositories.
- Describe how to perform quality control testing of lozenges, troches, sticks, and suppositories.
- Select appropriate packaging for the compounded lozenges, troches, sticks, and suppositories.
- Define the labeling requirements for lozenges, troches, sticks, and suppositories.
- Evaluate the stability of lozenges, troches, sticks, and suppositories.

INTRODUCTION

Lozenges, troches, sticks, and suppositories are all solid dosage forms that are prepared similarly by using molds. Each is designed to melt, soften, or dissolve at body temperature upon administration.

Types and Definitions

Lozenges and troches are both oral dosage forms that are placed in the oral cavity, either onto the tongue or into the cheek pouch, and usually meant to **disintegrate** over time. Recently, soft, chewable troches have been developed and are intended to be chewed and swallowed, delivering medication in the gastrointestinal track. Sticks are prepared for the topical use of either medications or cosmetics. Suppositories are used to deliver medications via the rectum, the vagina, or the urethra. All of these dosage forms are prepared by using molds, and calculations for calibration of the mold are the same. However, since some of the applications and methods of preparation vary, each will be discussed individually.

disintegrate
to decompose or break down

troche
interchangeable term with lozenges, but sometimes made in soft form

LOZENGES AND TROCHES

The terms *lozenge* and **troche** are often used interchangeably. However, there is one distinct difference between the two. A lozenge is never chewed and swallowed, but is placed in the oral cavity to dissolve slowly over time. Historically, troches were meant to be used in the same way. Recently, however, soft and chewable troches have been developed. These newer forms of troches can be placed in the mouth to dissolve, or they may be chewed and swallowed. How troches are used will depend on the medication and how it is to be delivered, as determined by the prescriber. Either a lozenge or a troche may be used when the treatment is intended for either a local effect by bathing the oral cavity and throat, or a systemic effect by absorption through mucousal tissues or by way of the gastrointestinal tract.

In the past, lozenges and troches, because of the length of time they stayed in the mouth, were used for the relief of minor sore throat pain or irritations in the mouth. They were used extensively to deliver antiseptics and anesthetics to the oral cavity. Today, however, lozenges and troches are being compounded with the specific patient in mind for a wide variety of drug classes. A few common drug classes prepared in the form of a lozenge or troche include antimicrobials, analgesics, antitussives, astringents, corticosteroids, decongestants, and demulcents.

Lozenges and troches may be considered as an alternative dosage form in many instances. As mentioned earlier, a lozenge or troche may be recommended when the desired effect is to release the active ingredient slowly, or directly into **mucosal tissue** as opposed to releasing the medication in the gastrointestinal tract. This dosage form may also be used when a patient has difficulty swallowing other oral dosage forms such as tablets or capsules. They may be substituted for an oral liquid dose when there is damage or weakness to the tongue and throat muscles that may cause choking with the liquid medication, such as with the stroke victim.

mucosal tissue
membrane tissue lining all body passages that communicate with the air

Some of the advantages to using troches are that they are easy to handle, their excipients have a demulcent effect, and they are easy to administer to a variety of patients. Patient types that may benefit from the use of troches include pediatrics, geriatrics, and hospice patients. Since their base is made of sugar, troches generally have a pleasant taste, which makes them a popular choice. They can be compounded extemporaneously quite easily with a minimal amount of equipment. However, their preparation does require a moderate amount of labor and time.

WORKPLACE WISDOM

One disadvantage to the troche form is that it could be mistaken for candy, especially by a child. Patients or caregivers should be warned to keep these and all medications out of the reach of children. They should also be cautioned against associating the medicated troche with candy.

STICKS

Medicated sticks are a unique solid dosage form used in topical application of local anesthetics, sunscreens, antivirals, antibiotics, and, of course, cosmetics. Although cosmetic sticks are viewed as tools to improve appearance, they also may contain pharmaceutical active ingredients that serve to heal or protect. For example, a lip balm, which moisturizes the lips, may contain both an antiviral and a sunscreen for use in the treatment and prevention of a herpes simplex outbreak. Sticks offer patients, physicians, and pharmacists a unique dosage form that is convenient, relatively stable, and fairly easy to prepare. Although relatively simple, the process of properly preparing sticks can be a bit time consuming.

It is imperative that the final product be pharmaceutically elegant and acceptable to the patient using it. Sticks should not be so hard that they crumble upon application; nor should they be so greasy that they smear when applied. Likewise, a stick should not be so soft that it liquefies upon application, resulting in the medication running off the affected area. Depending on the application site, the stick's consistency should be such that it delivers the medication easily and smoothly, completely coating the affected area with an appropriate amount of the drug being used to treat or protect.

SUPPOSITORIES

Suppositories are a solid dosage form used to administer medication by way of the rectum, the vagina, or the urethral tract. They are meant to melt or undergo dissolution at body temperature, delivering the needed drug either locally or **systemically**. The route of delivery and the particular patient will determine the shape and size of the suppository. The amount of medication incorporated into the suppository will also be a determining factor for weight.

systemically
of or relating to systemic circulation

Rectal suppositories are conical or cylindrical in shape. They are tapered at either one end or both ends for ease of insertion. Adult suppositories typically weigh approximately 2 gm and are anywhere from one inch long to one and a half inches long. Infant suppositories are usually about half the size of adult suppositories.

Vaginal suppositories are available in a variety of shapes. They may be conical, cylindrical, globular, ovoid, or some other shape. They usually weigh between 3 gm and 5 gm each. Vaginal suppositories are most commonly made from water soluble bases such as polyethylene glycols or glycerinated gelatin, as these bases help to minimize leakage. Another form of vaginal suppository is one that is made by using a gelatin capsule such as for Boric Acid. The gelatin will melt or decompose in bodily fluids and thus release the enclosed medication. One other form of vaginal suppository is the compressed tablet, which is also known as an insert.

Urethral suppositories are pencil shaped with a 5 mm diameter. The length of the suppository will vary depending on the gender of the patient. The urethral suppository designed for a female is 50 mm in length and weighs approximately 2 gm. For males, the suppository is 125 mm in length and weighs about 4 gm. Urethral suppositories are rarely prescribed.

Manufactured molds are available for compounding urethral suppositories, but a straw or thin glass tube can be used as well. A 1-ml topical or tuberculin syringe will also work. The tip of the syringe should be removed with a razor blade or a pencil sharpener. A syringe type mold is filled by putting the melted base into a 10-ml topical syringe and filling the 1-ml syringe from the back. The urethral suppository can be removed from this type of mold by inserting the warmed plunger into the syringe, gently applying pressure to the plunger until the suppository has been fully expelled.

Suppositories can be used for either a local effect or a systemic effect. The most commonly prescribed suppositories are for a local effect, such as soothing irritated tissues or to stimulate defecation. Local applications include the treatment of hemorrhoids, itching, and infections. Introduction of medication into the vagina may result in systemic effects. Circulatory system absorption may be exerted through the urethra or the rectum as well.

Suppositories are especially useful for the patient who cannot swallow, where a particular drug may not be tolerated orally, or when the pH and/or enzymes of the gastrointestinal tract will inactivate the needed medication. They are also useful for administering medications to infants and small children, severely debilitated patients, and in the instance where a parenteral route may not be appropriate. A variety of drugs for systemic absorption may be administered by way of a suppository. These include antinauseants, asthma medications, analgesics, and hormones.

Composition and Ingredients

There are many ingredients and methods of composition when compounding lozenges, troches, sticks and suppositories.

LOZENGES AND TROCHES

Hard troches, or lozenges, are made of a hard candy base consisting of sugars and other carbohydrates, such as corn syrup. They will generally have an adhesive agent, such as acacia, added. Hard troches are usually placed in the mouth, either on the tongue or into the cheek pouch, and are meant to dissolve without being chewed. Troches, which are not necessarily hard, may also be intended to dissolve. These troches are made from bases such as Fattibase® or other polyethyline glycols (PEGs).

Chewable troches may be either soft or firm and are meant to be chewed and swallowed. Recently, soft chewable troches have become more popular in treating young patients. One type of soft chewable troche is made from a gelatin base, resulting in a "gummy" type of product.

Chewable troches, whether soft or firm, may be made from a variety of different bases, including a peanut butter and hydrogenated vegetable mixture, chocolate mixed with a hydrogenated vegetable solid, polyethyline glycols, gelatin, and other similar materials. Which base is most appropriate will depend on the patient, the symptoms being treated, the active ingredient or needed excipients, the desired effect of the medication, solubility of the active ingredient, stability of the active ingredient (some drugs may be heat-sensitive), the size of the dose being incorporated, and certain other factors that may come into play. All these things should be considered before deciding on the best recommendation for dosage form.

STICKS

Materials used in preparing medicated sticks include waxes, polymers, resins, dry solids fused into a firm mass, and fused crystals (See Table 6-1). The type of stick being made is determined by the materials being used. Essentially, there are three types of sticks extemporaneously compounded for medicinal use: hard

TABLE 6-1 Ingredients Used to Prepare Medicated Sticks

Ingredient	Notes
Castor oil	has a high viscosity that will prevent settling of solid ingredients and will lessen the tendency of runoff upon application.
Cocoa butter	popular because it will melt at body temperature. However, it has a tendency to produce a finished product with improper consistency.
Vegetable oils	like corn oil, olive oil, or sesame oil, may turn rancid.
Mineral oils	resist rancidity, but have a limited ability to dissolve some ingredients.
Petrolatum	is very stable and produces a glossy finish.
Lanolin and other absorption bases	will aid in incorporating aqueous-based products.
Lecithin	is helpful for improving texture and application.
Carnauba wax	in a small percentage, will raise the melting point and add strength to the finished product.
Candelilla wax	has a low melting point and must be used in large quantities to obtain proper effects.
Beeswax	is a stiffening agent. It should not be used as the sole wax, as a dull stick that is difficult to apply will result.
Paraffin waxes	are weak and brittle, but in small amounts may enhance glossiness.

sticks, soft opaque sticks, and soft clear sticks. Hard sticks consist of crystalline powders that are fused by heat or held together with a binder such as cocoa butter or petrolatum. An example of the hard stick is the styptic pencil. Soft opaque sticks will usually contain petrolatum, cocoa butter, and PEGs in their base; most medication sticks are of this type. An example of the soft opaque stick is a lip balm containing acyclovir and a sunscreen. Soft clear sticks are made from sodium stearate and propylene glycol and usually contain water or alcohol. The most common example of the soft clear stick is the deodorant stick.

SUPPOSITORIES

Bases used in compounding suppositories should be stable, nonirritating, and both chemically and physiologically inactive. They should melt or dissolve in the body cavity where they are inserted. A properly chosen base will not bind or otherwise interfere with the release or absorption of the active ingredient contained within. The base should enable a product to be made that is esthetically acceptable to the patient. The drug to be incorporated will also affect the desirable characteristics of a suppository. For example, some drugs may lower the melting point of a base; therefore, a base with a higher melting point should be used. Climate is another consideration in determining the most appropriate base. A base with a higher melting point would be recommended if the suppository is dispensed in a tropical area.

There are many bases and additives to choose from that will enhance the final product when compounding suppositories (see Table 6-2). Before choosing an appropriate base, one must consider several factors, including patient sensitivities to certain ingredients, drug–base compatibility, solubility, stability,

TABLE 6-2 Commonly Used Bases for Suppositories

Base	Characteristics
Fattibase®	a solid, opaque-white, preblended base made of triglycerides derived from palm, palm kernel, and coconut oils, with self-emulsifying agents. It is stable with a low imitation profile, needs no special storage requirements, is uniform in composition, and has a bland taste and controlled melting range. It will readily release from a mold; therefore, mold lubrication is not necessary. Its melting point is 35–37°C and the specific gravity is 0.89 at 37°C.
Polybase®	a solid, white, preblended base that is made up of a homogeneous mixture of PEGs and polysorbate 80. It is water-miscible and is stable at room temperature. Its specific gravity is 1.177 at 25°C. It does not require mold lubrication.
Cocoa butter	a solid, oil-based product that softens at 30°C and melts at 34°C. One disadvantage to using cocoa butter as a suppository base is its tendency to leak from the body cavity as it is immiscible with body fluids. Suppositories made from cocoa butter will release easily from the molds only if the molds are absolutely clean and dry, and the cocoa butter has not been overheated. The percentage for solids contained in a cocoa butter base should not exceed 30 percent as brittleness may result. Fracturing of cocoa butter suppositories may also occur from shock cooling. This can be avoided if the temperature of the mold is close to the temperature of the melted base. An addition of 2 percent or less of castor oil, glycerin, or propylene glycol will lessen the brittleness of the base and make it more pliable.
Glycerin bases	composed of 91 percent glycerin, 9 percent sodium stearate, and 5 percent purified water. Glycerin suppositories should be stored in air-tight containers, as they are hygroscopic. Glycerin suppositories are not recommended for rectal use, but are occasionally used to prepare vaginal suppositories.

desired rate of release of the drug, total amount of drug and/or excipients to be incorporated, and whether a local effect or systemic effect is preferred by the prescriber. A few of the most commonly used suppository bases are Fattibase®, Polybase®, cocoa butter, and glycerin bases.

Preparation and Compounding Techniques

There are many steps in the preparation and compounding of lozenges, troches, sticks and suppositories.

LOZENGES AND TROCHES

Many different molds are available for the compounding of troches. No matter which mold is used, it must be calibrated for each formula. This is done by filling a sampling of 10 molds with the base only, allowing the troches to set, removing them from the mold, and then weighing each one. A total weight of all the troches contained in the sample should also be performed. The total weight is then divided by the number of troches contained in the sample, resulting in an average weight for each. This figure will be used when performing the calculations for the amount of base to be used in the formula.

There may or may not be a displacement factor, depending on the physical characteristics of the active ingredient or excipients and the total amount of powders being incorporated into the base. This figure will vary with each medication being formulated. As a general rule, solid ingredients will displace the base anywhere from 70 to 90 percent. Liquid ingredients will have a displacement value of 100 percent.

It is usually necessary to prepare the molds beforehand by spraying them lightly with a food-grade, nonstick cooking spray. The cavity plate as well as the base plate should be coated and then set on a paper towel to drain. Lubricating the molds will allow the troches to be removed easily without breaking or sticking to the mold cavities or base plate.

The powder ingredients listed in the formula are mixed together in geometric proportion, using a mortar and pestle. The powder mixture is then passed through a sieve to reduce the particles and to ensure a uniform size of the particles throughout the final product.

Hard candy troches are usually prepared by heating the sugars and syrup to a proper temperature. The temperature will vary with each formula, but is usually around 154°C. When the desired temperature has been reached, the base is removed from the heat. The powder mixture is added in increments with stirring, **incorporating** the active ingredient and other excipients. Flavoring and coloring agents are added next and again stirred until the color is uniform. The mixture is then poured into the pre-calibrated molds.

incorporating
uniting with

Another method for making hard troches is to pour out the mixture onto a prepared surface and stretch the mass into a ribbon; the ribbon is then cut into equal pieces. Extreme care must be taken to ensure that the pieces are of equal size and weight so that the correct dosage is contained within each piece.

Soft and chewable troches are prepared similarly, using the following methods: The appropriate base is measured out and melted in a hot water bath at 55°C. This can be accomplished by putting some hot water into a 1000 ml beaker and then lowering a 400 ml beaker inside of it.

WORKPLACE WISDOM

Glass beads can be placed between the beakers to prevent the beakers from knocking into one another.

The beakers are then placed onto a hot plate that has been set on medium. The base is placed into the inner beaker to be melted. Care must be taken not to overheat the base, resulting in ruining the base or causing degradation of the active ingredient. A thermometer should be used during this part of the compounding procedure. Some sweeteners are heat sensitive as well, and this should be taken into consideration. It is recommended that a microwave not be used for melting the base, as it is too easy to overheat and the base will not always melt consistently.

Regardless of which troche is being compounded, there are three ingredients that are usually used in the same proportion for all formulations. Silica gel is used as a suspending agent, acacia is used as a firming agent, and sweetening agents, such as acesulfame, Nutrasweet, stevia, or saccharin are added. This portion of the formula is often called the troche mix. The troche mix is then comminuted with the active ingredient by using a mortar and pestle and applying the principle of geometric proportion.

After the powders have been thoroughly mixed, they are sifted through a sieve of 100 mesh size into the liquefied base. This will ensure uniform particle size throughout the final product. A plastic spatula should be used to do this, as a metal one may impart metal shavings from the sieve into the base. Next, the mixture should be stirred to completely and evenly suspend all the ingredients.

The mixture is then removed from the hot plate, and coloring and/or flavoring agents are added. Flavoring agents are generally calculated at a range of 0.05 ml to 0.65 ml per 26 troches, depending on the chemical taste you are trying to mask and the vehicle used in the formula. Coloring and flavoring agents are added only at the completion of the formula, since many of these agents are heat sensitive and will degrade if left on the heat source too long. Again, the mixture should be thoroughly stirred to evenly incorporate the flavors and colors throughout (Figure 6-1 A-E).

When the color is uniform, the mixture is ready to be poured into the prepared molds. The preparer must work somewhat quickly to get the mixture poured before it begins to harden. However, working too quickly may result in air pockets being formed in the troche. It may be necessary to return the mixture to the heat source momentarily to soften if it becomes too hard to pour. Experience with this procedure will help the preparer become familiar with the most efficient technique.

When all the liquid has been poured into the troche mold, the liquid should be pushed around the top of the mold, moving the overflow of the base from some cavities into cavities that are not completely full. This can be done by using an angled spatula or a plastic powder scraper. When the cavities are completely and evenly filled, they should be examined for uniformity of fill. Depending on the consistency of the final product, it may be necessary to "burp" the troches. This is done by lightly tapping the mold on a hard surface.

Pits or recessed areas may form as the troches begin to set. This can be rectified in one of two ways. First, a heat gun, or small hand-held hair dryer,

Figure 6-1
Compounding troches

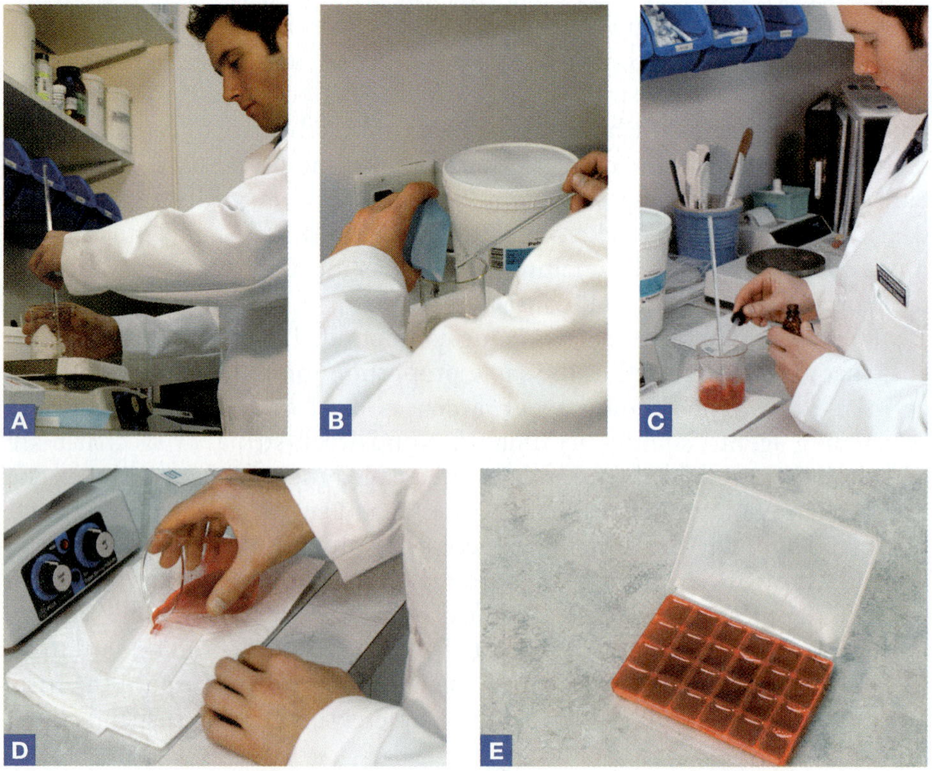

may be used to slightly melt the tops of the troches. The melted liquid is then moved around to fill in the recessed areas. The second method involves using a metal spatula that has been heated in hot water. The hot spatula will melt the top layer of the troches and allow the preparer to move the melted liquid into the pitted areas. Even if the troches look evenly filled upon examination, one of these procedures should be performed in order to "polish" the tops of the troches. This will result in a product that is pharmaceutically elegant.

STICKS

Extreme care must be taken when preparing medication sticks. It is imperative that a quality product is produced in order for the stick to be both acceptable and usable. A stick should spread easily onto the application site without excessive greasiness. A stick should be uniform throughout, and it should be stable. It is likewise important the stick not crumble, crack, sweat, or **mottle**.

mottle
to mark with spots or blotches

In order to prepare a good stick, one must be familiar with the physical characteristics of the waxes and other vehicles used for preparation. Some waxes such as carnauba have a high melting point, whereas others such as beeswax, paraffin, and cocoa butter have relatively low melting points. Certain excipients included in the formula should be considered also. For example, fatty acids such as stearic acid and fatty alcohols such as cetyl alcohol and stearyl alcohol are commonly used and have unique melting or congealing points. Polyethyline glycols (PEGs) are water soluble and thus are easily removed from the skin.

Sticks are not made from one waxy substance alone; several ingredients are required to produce a desirable product. The high melting point waxes must be blended with the low melting point waxes to produce a product that will melt or soften at body temperature. Lubricants are necessary to aid in spreading of the medicated stick as well as to minimize coherence of the waxes. Proper balance of these ingredients is necessary in order to develop a stick that will have the physical properties needed for an efficacious and desirable product. The end result should be a medication stick that melts at body temperature and contains the lubricants and other excipients that promote absorption as well as emollient effects.

The consistency of the stick is determined by the melting point of the waxes in the formula. To change the consistency of the final product, the percentage of the wax with the highest melting point is increased or decreased so that its melting point is adjusted.

It is important to be familiar with the different ingredients and their physical properties used in formulating medication sticks. Each ingredient may offer an advantage or a disadvantage, depending on its physical characteristics (see Table 6-3).

Sticks are usually prepared by using some type of mold. It may be a mold that has been manufactured specifically for this purpose. Alternatively, a mold can be made by using an item already in the compounding pharmacy such as a 1 ml topical syringe that has had the tip cut off or possibly a suppository mold.

In some cases, such as when preparing hard sticks, it may be necessary to lubricate the mold prior to preparation. This will allow the hard stick to be removed from the mold without breaking or sticking. Since soft opaque and soft clear sticks usually contain lubricants and waxes, this step is not necessary for these types of sticks.

TABLE 6-3 Compounding Hints for Medication Sticks

- Vitamins E and A will enhance the emollient and skin conditioning effects.
- Zinc oxide or PABA will act as a sunblock.
- Flavoring agents added to lip balms will please the user and thus possibly ensure compliancy. Likewise, perfume oils may be added to topical skin preparations, reducing a possible offensive odor.

As discussed earlier, the mold must be calibrated for each formula being prepared. The total amount of ingredients contained in the formula will determine whether a displacement factor must be used when calculating the amount of base needed. To calibrate the mold, a sample of 10 sticks is prepared, using the base alone. Each stick is then weighed individually and the weight recorded. The sample batch is then weighed as a whole and the total weight divided by the number of sticks contained in the sample. This figure represents the average weight of each stick. The individual weight is multiplied by the number of sticks to be made. The solid ingredients are calculated and then subtracted from the base amount, either in its entirety or a percentage, depending on the physical characteristics of the active ingredient and/or excipients. The total amount of the excipients will also be a factor in determining displacement.

The powders to be used in the formula are mixed in geometric proportion. The bases used in the formula are melted at the appropriate temperature and then mixed together. When the base is liquefied, the solids can be thoroughly mixed in by stirring. Finally, coloring and flavoring agents are added if necessary, and the mixture is stirred until uniform. The mixture is then poured into the molds and left to set. Each stick should be examined for solidity and proper finish (Figure 6-2 A-E).

SUPPOSITORIES

Suppositories can be prepared several ways, including hand molding, fusion, or compression. When extemporaneously compounding suppositories, either hand molding or fusion is most commonly used (see Table 6-4).

Hand molding suppositories requires considerable skill that is achieved with experience. This method allows for the suppository to be formed without the use of heat, which is appropriate when a drug is heat labile. Generally, this method is performed when using cocoa butter as the base, as it has a low melting point and can be shaped and manipulated at room temperature. The preparer should wear plastic gloves during the forming process. The cocoa butter is grated, weighed, and then mixed with the active ingredient with the use of a mortar and pestle. When the mixture becomes a solid form, it can be shaped with the hands into a long cylinder. It is then cut into the desired length, and the tip is rounded. Each prepared suppository should be equal in size and weight, ensuring that the exact required dose is contained within.

fusion
the merging of different elements

Fusion is a method whereby the base is melted by using a water bath on a hotplate and poured into pre-calibrated molds. The molds should be inspected for cleanliness and dryness prior to use. Determination as to whether

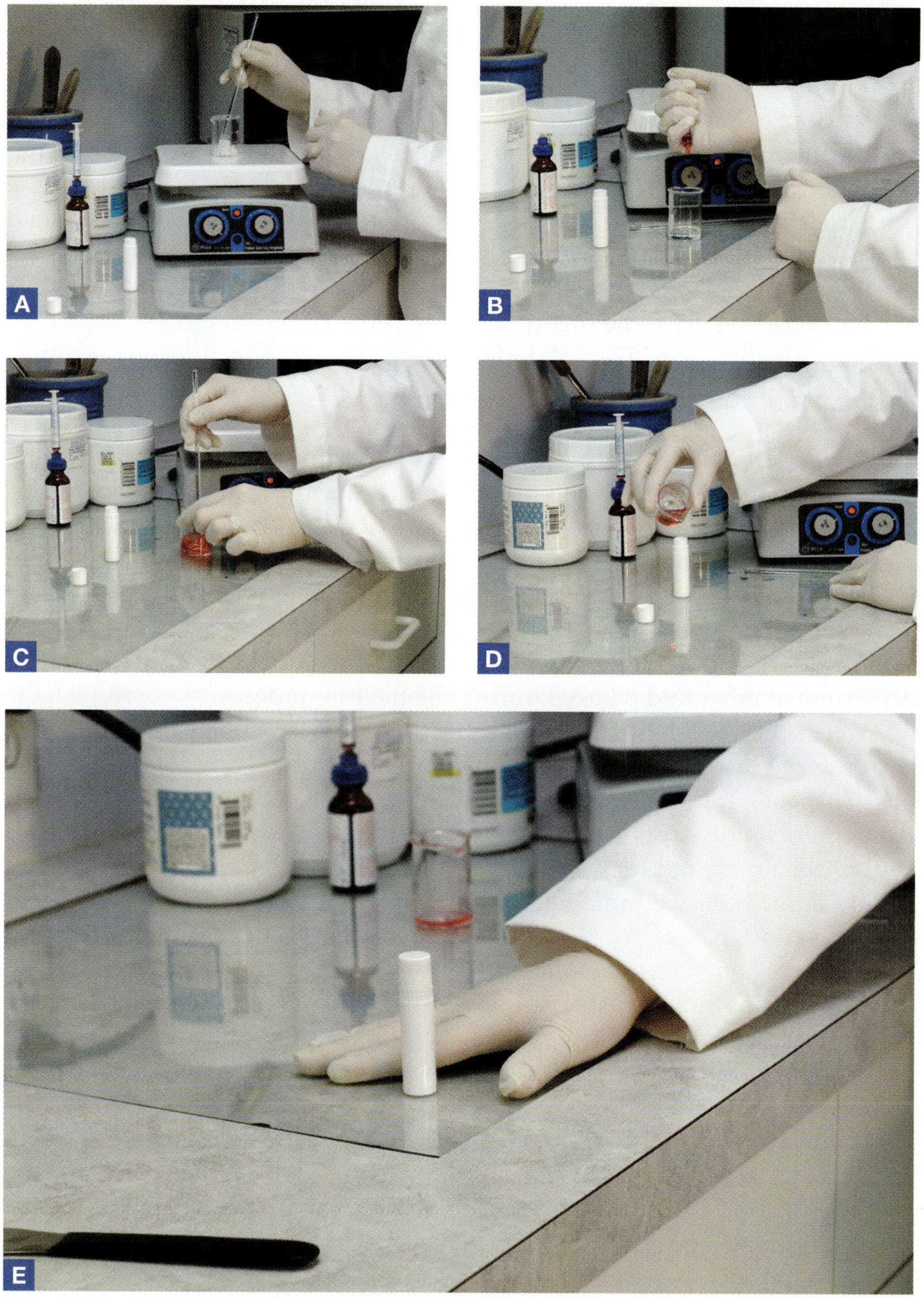

Figure 6-2
Compounding a medicated stick

a lubricant is necessary should be made beforehand and applied as necessary. Molds should be at room temperature at the time of filling.

When the base is completely liquefied, the active ingredient and excipients are added with stirring. When all the ingredients have been thoroughly mixed in the base, it is poured into the molds and left to cool and set. Once the pouring process has begun it should not be interrupted, as a layered effect will occur, resulting in weakness that will cause the suppository to separate. The mold cavities should be slightly overfilled to allow for contraction during

WORKPLACE WISDOM

When working with suppository molds, it may be advisable to slightly heat the molds prior to filling, bringing their temperature more closely to that of the melted base.

TABLE 6-4 Equipment Required to Compound Suppositories

Suppository molds
Water bath, hotplate
Thermometer
Beakers
Glass stirring rods
Tongs
Grater
Spatula
Foil suppository wraps
Cardboard sleeves

the cooling process. When the suppositories are cooled and hardened, the excess is trimmed by using a clean single-edge razor or a heated spatula. The suppositories should be examined for uniformity of fill and for any recessed areas that may have formed.

Excipients used in compounding suppositories will vary from formula to formula. Depending on the base used and the physical characteristics of the drug to be incorporated, it may be necessary to use a suspending agent such as acacia or silica gel. Other times, the active ingredient will be the only powder to be incorporated.

Powders that are to be incorporated into the suppository base should be in an impalpable form. The solid ingredients are mixed in geometric proportion and then passed through a sieve to ensure uniform particle size throughout the mixture.

The base is melted with a hot water bath. This can be done by putting some hot water into a 1000 ml beaker and then putting a 400 ml beaker inside the larger beaker. Glass beads can be used between the beakers to prevent them from knocking into one another. The base to be melted is placed in the 400 ml beaker, and both beakers are put on a hot plate set to medium heat. Extreme care must be taken to avoid overheating. Overheating the base may result in ruining the base or degrading the medicinal agent to be added. A thermometer should be used during the melting process.

When the base has turned to liquid, the powder ingredients are added with thorough stirring. When the powder mixture has completely dissolved or is suspended, the melt is poured into the molds and left to cool at room temperature. The suppositories are completely cooled when the mold feels cool to the touch and no warmth is present. The hot or warm suppositories should never be placed in a refrigerator or freezer to cool. This could result in shock cooling, which will cause the suppositories to crack and may also cause them to stick to the mold.

In preparing suppositories, it is always advisable to prepare 10 percent excess to allow for loss during preparation and for overfilling. The cavities should be overfilled to allow for contraction during cooling. Contraction of the base as it cools will result in the suppositories removing easily from the mold, but may also cause a depression to form in the back end of the suppository at the opening of the mold cavity. When the suppositories have sufficiently cooled, the excess is scraped off. Any divots that may have form can be filled by taking a small amount of the excess and rubbing it in a circular motion into the crevice until the top is full and smooth (Figure 6-3 A-D).

Quality Control

All compounding activities should include double checks on all weights or measurements and documentation of all steps, weight or measurements, calculations, and end-product testing, as part of a good quality assurance program. Quality control and end-product testing should include checking the final volume or weight of the compounded product, appearance (including uniform color), odor, and pH.

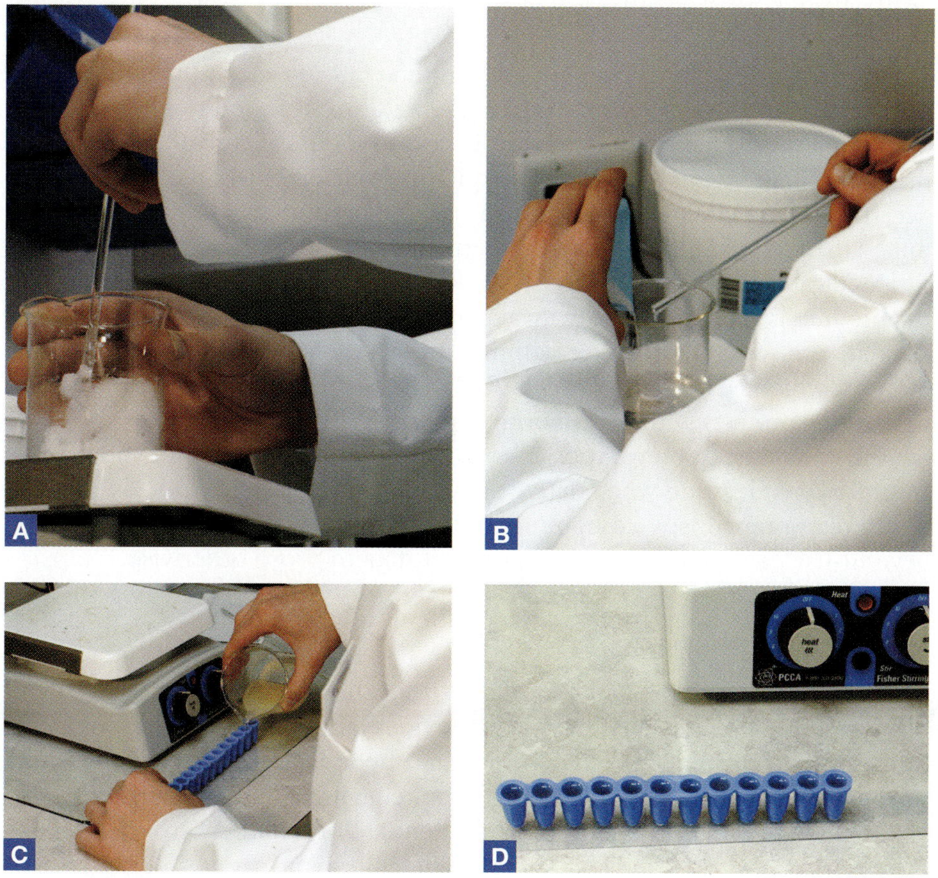

Figure 6-3
Compounding suppositories

Packaging

Finished suppositories should be individually wrapped in foil papers available for this purpose. Wrapped suppositories may be placed in wide mouth containers or cardboard slides. They may also be dispensed in the disposable mold in which they were prepared. If the latter method is used, the recipient should be shown how to properly remove the suppository without breaking it. Proper packaging for dispensing is important, as improper packaging may result in breakage, deformation, or staining of the finished product. Suppositories made from PEG bases should not be stored or dispensed in polysterene prescription vials, as the polyethyline glycol will adversely interact with the polysterene. All PEG-based suppositories should be stored and dispensed in either glass or cardboard containers.

Labeling

The following information should be included on all compounding labels: generic or chemical name of the active ingredient(s), strength or quantity, an assigned pharmacy lot number, beyond-use or expiration dating, storage requirements, and instructions for use.

Stability

Finished lozenges and troches are dry and therefore are generally stable as long as they are protected from heat and moisture. Lozenges and troches prepared from a manufactured product should have a beyond-use date of 25 percent of the time remaining on the product's expiration or six months, whichever is earlier. If a USP/NF chemical powder is used, the beyond-use date is six months unless there is evidence to support alternate dating for the product.

Medication sticks are generally stable as long as they are stored properly. If the product is compounded by means of manufactured products, the beyond-use date is 25 percent of the remaining time on the product's expiration or six months, whichever is earlier. If USP/NF ingredients are used, it is appropriate to label the product with a six-month expiry unless evidence proves otherwise. Since heat is used in preparation of these products, the formulator should take this into consideration when determining a beyond-use date.

Extemporaneously compounded suppositories will generally have a beyond-use date of 30 days unless there is data to prove otherwise.

Patient Counseling

The patient or caregiver should be asked if he or she would like counseling about the compound from the pharmacist. Instructions for use, including how often the drug is taken, the duration of therapy, and the importance of completing the entire therapy, as well as any pertinent storage requirements, should be expressed.

It is important to mention the potential for children to mistake the lozenges/troches for candy and what guidelines for parents or custodians should be followed. Storage recommendation for lozenges and troches may be either at room temperature or refrigerated, depending on the active ingredient and the base used in the formula. They should not be exposed to a temperature greater than that of room temperature, as they may soften or melt. They should be stored in airtight containers to prevent drying out. Hard candy lozenges are especially hygroscopic and are prone to absorption of moisture in the air. It may be wise to recommend storing the package in a zipper bag, which will help to keep air away from the product.

The patient or caregiver should be given instructions to protect the product from moisture and heat when storing medication sticks.

Suppositories should be protected from heat and are usually stored in the refrigerator to preserve the active ingredient and prevent the base from softening. Instructions for the patient or the patient's caregiver should be included on the prescription label, along with directions to remove the outer wrapping, lubricate with white petrolatum or KY Jelly® or other appropriate product if necessary, and insert the suppository into the appropriate body cavity.

SUMMARY

Lozenges, troches, sticks, and suppositories provide numerous opportunities for the compounding pharmacy to meet the needs of the individual patient. Each dosage form requires specific procedures and techniques that will be perfected with practice.

PROFILES OF PRACTICE

Sample Formula: Powder Sugar-Based Troches

for training purposes only

Powder sugar	10 g
Lactose	1 g
Acacia	0.7 g
Purified water	qs

1. Accurately measure each ingredient.
2. Mix the acacia and purified water together to create a mucilage.
3. Sift the powder sugar and lactose together and slowly add enough mucilage to create an appropriate consistency.
4. Roll the product into a cylinder shape, and cut into 10 equal sections.
5. Allow to air dry, package, and label.

Sample Formula: Lip Balm

for training purposes only

Lactose NF Hydrous	0.2 g
Silica gel Micronized	0.12 g
Polyglycol 4500 MW, NF	6.5 g
Polyglycol 300 MW, NF	15 ml

1. Accurately measure each ingredient.
2. Melt the polyglycol 4500 and polyglycol 300 together on a hot plate until the solution is clear.
3. Triturate the lactose and silica gel together in a small mortar.
4. Sift the powders into the melted base solution.
5. Turn off heat and mix.
6. Add color and/or flavoring.
7. Pour into lip balm tubes and label (makes 4).

Sample Formula: Suppositories

for training purposes only

Lactose	1 mg
Silica gel	20 mg
Fatty acid base	qs

1. Accurately measure each ingredient.
2. Melt the fatty acid base on a hot plate.
3. Sift the powders into the melted base solution.
4. Turn off heat and mix.
5. Pour into molds, then refrigerate to harden.
6. Package and label.

PROFILES OF PRACTICE

CHAPTER TERMS

disintegrate
to decompose or break down

fusion
the merging of different elements

incorporating
uniting with

mottle
to mark with spots or blotches

mucosal tissue
membrane tissue lining all body passages that communicate with the air

systemically
of or relating to systemic circulation

troche
interchangeable term with lozenges, but sometimes made in soft form

CHAPTER 6

CHAPTER REVIEW QUESTIONS

1. Which of the following is not a type of medicated stick that can be compounded for oral administration?
   a. hard
   b. chewable
   c. soft clear
   d. soft opaque
2. What is the end result desired when preparing medication sticks?
   a. uniform
   b. greasy
   c. mottled
   d. cracked
3. By what route of delivery can one administer suppositories?
   a. rectal
   b. vaginal
   c. urethral
   d. all of the above
4. Which of the following would be more suited to be compounded as a lozenge or troche?
   a. antitussives
   b. anti-infective
   c. antiviral
   d. anti-itch
5. Which ingredient used in the preparation of medicated sticks is very stable and produces a glossy finish?
   a. cocoa butter
   b. carnauba wax
   c. petrolatum
   d. vegetable oil
6. True or false: As a general rule, when compounding troches, one should assume that liquid ingredients will displace 70%–90% and solid ingredients will displace 100%.
   a. true
   b. false
7. True or false: The term "systemic" relates to circulation.
   a. true
   b. false
8. List six pieces of equipment to compound suppositories.
9. List a situation for which a medicated stick would be an appropriate choice for the delivery of a medicinal agent.
10. **Critical Thinking** Describe the caution that should be taken when dispensing lozenges or troches to households with children.

Resources and References

1. Allen, Loyd V. Jr., Ph.D. *The Art, Science, and Technology of Pharmaceutical Compounding*. Washington, DC: American Pharmaceutical Association, 1998.
2. *Remington's Pharmaceutical Sciences*, 15th Edition. Easton, PA: Mack Publishing Co., 1975.
3. Allen, Loyd V. Jr., Ph.D., *Secundum Artem: Compounding Suppositories, Part I*. Vol. 3, No. 3, Minneapolis, MN.
4. Allen, Loyd V. Jr., Ph.D. , *Secundum Artem: Compounding Suppositories, Part II*. Vol. 3, No. 4, Minneapolis, MN.

CHAPTER 7

Solutions, Suspensions, and Emulsions

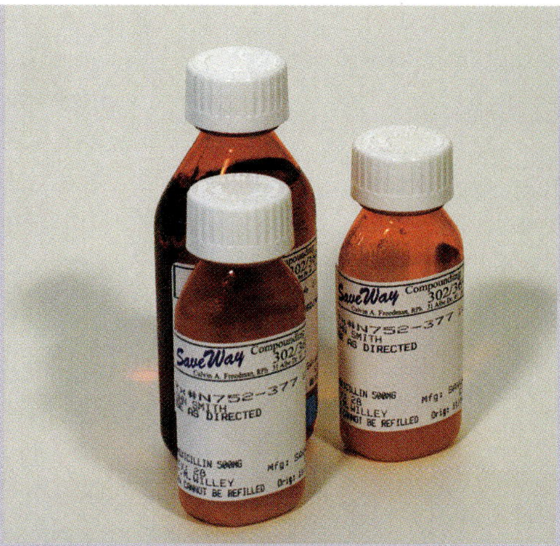

Learning Objectives

After completing this chapter, you should be able to:

- Distinguish the different types of solutions, suspensions, and emulsions.
- List the ingredients and composition properties required to prepare solutions, suspensions, and emulsions.
- Explain the procedures and techniques used to prepare solutions, suspensions, and emulsions.
- Describe how to perform quality control testing of solutions, suspensions, and emulsions.
- Select appropriate packaging for the compounded solutions, suspensions, and emulsions.
- Define the labeling requirements for solutions, suspensions, and emulsions.
- Evaluate the stability of solutions, suspensions, and emulsions in assigning beyond-use dates and storage requirements.

INTRODUCTION

Liquid compounds are probably the most commonly prepared compounds in a pharmacy. They can be administered by mouth, topically, rectally, vaginally, and in the eyes or ears. The most frequently prepared liquid dosage form is intended for oral administration. This chapter will focus on oral dosage forms; however, the preparation information is similar and can be applied to other liquid dosage forms.

Types and Definitions

There are many different reasons why liquid compounds need to be prepared. Many commercial drug products are not available as oral liquids, although there are several patient populations that need them: pediatric patients, some **geriatric** patients, patients with naso-gastric or gastric tubes, and patients who cannot swallow tablets or capsules.

SOLUTIONS

Solutions are clear liquid preparations in which all of the ingredients are miscible or dissolved in a suitable vehicle and may contain one or more active ingredients. There are five types of solutions: oral liquid solutions, topical solutions,

geriatric
referring to a senior patient

solutions
clear liquid preparations in which all of the ingredients are dissolved in a suitable vehicle; may contain one or more active ingredients

elixirs
solutions that are sweetened and alcohol-based

aromatic waters
clear, saturated aqueous solutions of volatile oils or aromatic substances; may be used internally or externally

suspensions
liquids that contain ingredients, both active and inert, that are not soluble in the vehicle, but rather suspended or resuspended upon shaking

emulsions
a type of suspension consisting of two immiscible liquids and an emulsifying agent to hold them together

syrups, elixirs, and aromatic waters. Concentrated sugar or sugar-substitute aqueous liquids are called syrups and are used to improve the taste of some foul- or bitter-tasting active ingredients. **Elixirs** are solutions that are sweetened and alcohol-based. They are primarily used for drugs that are soluble in alcohol then diluted with water. **Aromatic waters** are clear, saturated aqueous solutions of volatile oils or aromatic substances and may be used internally or externally.

SUSPENSIONS

Suspensions are liquids that contain ingredients, both active and inert, that are not soluble in the vehicle. They are two-phased systems consisting of fine solid particles dispersed in liquid, solid, or gas. Suspensions can either be applied topically or taken by mouth. Oral suspensions are generally prepared in a sweetened, flavored, and sometimes viscous vehicle. Topical suspensions are sometimes referred to as lotions.

EMULSIONS

An **emulsion** is a type of suspension consisting of two immiscible liquids and an emulsifying agent to hold them together. It consists of a dispersed or internal phase, a dispersion medium or external phase, and an emulsifying agent. There are two types of emulsions: water-in-oil (w/o) and oil-in-water (o/w). Generally, an emulsion intended for oral use is the oil-in-water type, whereas an emulsion intended for external use can be either. Water-in-oil emulsions are occlusive, greasy, and not water washable. Oil-in-water emulsions are water washable, hydrophilic, nonocclusive, and nongreasy, such as vanishing cream. Creams and lotions are examples of types of topical emulsions.

Composition and Ingredients

There are several factors that have to be considered when preparing any oral liquid: drug concentration and solubility, pH of the vehicle and pKa of the drug, taste, and stability.

SOLUTIONS

When considering solubility, it is important to know whether the drug is slightly soluble, soluble, or freely soluble—that is, to know how many milligrams of drug will dissolve in a precise number of milliliters of a specified vehicle. Usually, this information can be found in reference resources, such as *The Merck Index*, *USPDI*, or *Remington*, all of which should be part of any compounding pharmacy library. The important point to remember is that "like prefers like." For example, an acidic drug that is water soluble up to 500 mg/ml is going to be most stable in an acidic pH aqueous vehicle in a drug concentration below 500 mg/ml. If the pH increases to neutral or basic or the drug concentration exceeds 500 mg/ml, the liquid will become unstable and the drug may degrade and become inactive or precipitate out of the liquid. If a drug is not water soluble, but stable in an acidic pH, a suspending agent should be used to suspend the drug, then added to the vehicle in order to prepare the suspension. If a drug is an oil or lipophilic, an emulsion may be the best option.

Many drugs are bitter or have a bad taste or odor. Since pediatric patients receive a large number of these compounded oral liquids, taste is a very important factor in preparing oral liquids. A suspension or solution may be compounded that is very stable, but if it is not palatable and the child refuses to take it, the suspension or solution is not acceptable. Flavorings and sweeteners can be added to the preparations to overcome these problems, assuming that there will be no reaction either with the active ingredient or with the patient.

Other additives may be added to oral liquid compounds to make them more stable. Preservatives are added to prevent microbial contamination, since some of the aqueous vehicles are good growth media for bacteria. Research must be done before choosing a preservative to ensure that there is no problem either with the other ingredients or with the patient. Common preservatives used in oral liquids are listed in Table 7-1.

Other additives include antioxidants such as Butylated Hydroxytoluene, Vitamin C (or ascorbic acid), and Vitamin E, which prevent rancidity of oils or deterioration of other ingredients by inhibiting oxidation.

Buffers may be added to maintain the pH in a certain range for stability of the compound. Some drugs undergo oxidation, and an antioxidant, such as ascorbic acid, may be added to prevent this type of degradation.

buffers
ingredients that prevent change in the concentration of another chemical substance

Several vehicles are used for solutions, suspension, and emulsions. Oral solutions primarily use purified or distilled water, ethanol, glycerin, syrups, and blends of these different ingredients. A list of common syrups used for oral liquid compounds is shown in Table 7-2.

Although propylene glycol can also be found in oral solutions as a solvent, it is generally not desirable to use as the primary vehicle, especially in pediatrics, because of an increased seizure risk and an oral intake limit of 25 mg/kg per day set by the World Health Organization (WHO). Many of these same vehicles can be used in topical solutions. Other vehicles used in the preparation of compounded products to be used on the skin include acetone, isopropanol, propylene glycol, the polyethylene glycols (PEGs), collodion, many oils, numerous polymers, and sometime dimethyl sulfoxide (DMSO). Sterile topical solutions, such as ophthalmic, otic, and nasal preparations, require sterile water for injection, which is a higher purity grade of water.

SUSPENSIONS

Suspensions can be made from the same vehicles used to prepare solutions. Fixed oils, including vegetable oils such as sweet almond oil, corn oil, or peanut oil, may also be used as a suspending agent for some insoluble drug. Sodium

TABLE 7-1 Common Preservatives Used in Oral Liquid Compounds

Preservative	Concentration (%)
Ethyl Alcohol	15–20%
Benzoic Acid	0.1%
Methylparaben	≤ 0.2%
Propylparaben	≤ 0.2%
Sodium Benzoate	0.1%
Sorbic Acid	0.1%

TABLE 7-2 Common Syrup Vehicles Used in Oral Liquid Compounds

Syrup	pH	Alcohol Content (%)
Acacia Syrup	5.0	
Cherry Syrup	3.5–4.0	1–2
Coca-Cola™ Syrup	1.6–1.7	
Glycyrrhizia Syrup	6.0–6.5	5–6
Ora-Sweet®	4.0–4.5	
Ora-Sweet SF®	4.0–4.4	
Orange Syrup	2.5–3.0	2–5
Raspberry Syrup	3.0	1–2
Syrpalta™	4.5	
Simple Syrup, USP	6.5–7.0	

bicarbonate 8.4 percent for injection is necessary in the preparation of proton pump inhibitor (PPI) suspensions, such as omeprazole or lansoprazole suspensions, in order to create an environment of the proper pH. There are also commercial suspension vehicles, such as Ora-Plus® (Paddock Laboratories) and Suspendol-S®, available to simplify the compounding of suspensions. CaraCream® and ChocoBase® are commercial basic vehicles that can be used instead of the sodium bicarbonate 8.4 percent for injection to prepare the PPI suspensions. Table 7-3 lists the common suspending agents used in suspensions.

EMULSIONS

Emulsions contain three basic components: a lipid or oil phase, an aqueous phase, and the emulsifier. There are numerous emulsifiers that can be used in emulsions listed in Table 7-4. Common commercial emulsifiers include Methocel, PEG 400, and the Tweens and Spans.

Preparation and Compounding Techniques

Solutions are one of the easiest and most common liquids to compound.

SOLUTIONS

There are also a variety of different techniques that can be used to compound them. Most water soluble ingredients will dissolve in water by simply stirring, shaking, or allowing time to dissolve on their own. If the solution is

TABLE 7-3 Common Suspending Agents Used in Suspensions

Agent	Final Concentration (%)
Acacia, NF	2.0–5.0%
Carbomer Resins, NF	0.5–5.0%
Carboxymethylcellulose Sodium, USP	0.5–1.5%
Colloidal Silicon Dioxide, NF	1.5–3.5%
Methylcellulose, USP	0.5–5.0%
Tragacanth, NF	0.5–2.0%

TABLE 7-4 Emulsifiers and Stabilizers for Emulsions

Carbohydrates	**Surfactants**
Acacia	Anionic
Agar	Cationic
Pectin	Nonionic
Tragacanth	
Proteins	**Solids**
Casein	Aluminum hydroxide
Egg yolk	Bentonite
Gelatin	Magnesium hydroxide
High Molecular Weight Alcohols	
Cetyl alcohol	
Glyceryl monostearate	
Stearyl alcohol	

concentrated, heat may be needed to dissolve the ingredients while stirring. Other solutions may need a high degree of agitation, such as using a blender, to dissolve the ingredients. If commercial tablets are crushed and the active ingredient(s) is water soluble, the excipients from the tablets may be removed by filtration to clarify the solution. Other tips on compounding solutions can be found in Table 7-5.

ELIXIRS

Elixirs have a water component and an alcohol component as the vehicle. This is called **a co-solvent system**. When preparing an elixir, the alcohol-soluble ingredients should be dissolved in ethanol, and the water-soluble ingredients should be dissolved in water prior to mixing the two components together. When mixing the alcohol and water, it is necessary to stir constantly. The aqueous component should be added to the alcohol content while stirring to keep the alcohol concentration as high as possible.

co-solvent system
two ingredients together used as a solvent

WORKPLACE WISDOM
Remember that only ethanol should be used in oral elixirs, not isopropyl alcohol.

SUSPENSIONS

The first step in compounding a suspension is to reduce the particle size of the solid component of the suspension. This can be achieved in a variety of different ways. Grind the tablets or powder in a mortar with a pestle. Pass the

TABLE 7-5 Tips for Compounding Solutions and Syrups

1. Magnetic stirrers and electric mixers or blenders can save time compared with stirring rods and produce a more uniform product.
2. Using an ultrasonic bath can speed up the dissolution time of the ingredients in the vehicle.
3. When combining two liquids, the mixture should be constantly stirred to decrease the chance of incompatibilities due to concentrations.
4. Salts should be dissolved in a small amount of water before a viscous vehicle is added.
5. High-viscosity liquids should be added to low-viscosity liquids while constantly stirring.

powder ingredients through a 100 size mesh sieve. Tablets may be pulverized into a fine powder with a mortar and pestle, a coffee grinder or a tablet pulverizer attachment to a blender (Figure 7-1A-J).

hydrophilic
readily absorbing moisture

hydrophobic
property of repelling water

After the particle size is reduced, the fine powder should be wetted prior to mixing it with the primary vehicle. If the powder is **hydrophilic**, add a little water to it and mix until a paste is formed. If the powder is **hydrophobic**, add a little glycerin to it and mix until a paste is formed. Generally, a dry suspending agent should be wetted with glycerin, not water, to avoid clumping when adding the vehicle.

Slowly add the vehicle to the thick paste while constantly stirring. When the mixture is fluid, pour the mixture into a graduate and add the vehicle until the final, desired volume is achieved. The mixture should be poured into a beaker or back into the mortar and stirred again to achieve a uniform mixture. Homogenizers, manual or electric, can further reduce the solid particle size, smooth out any clumps in the suspension, and make a uniform suspension.

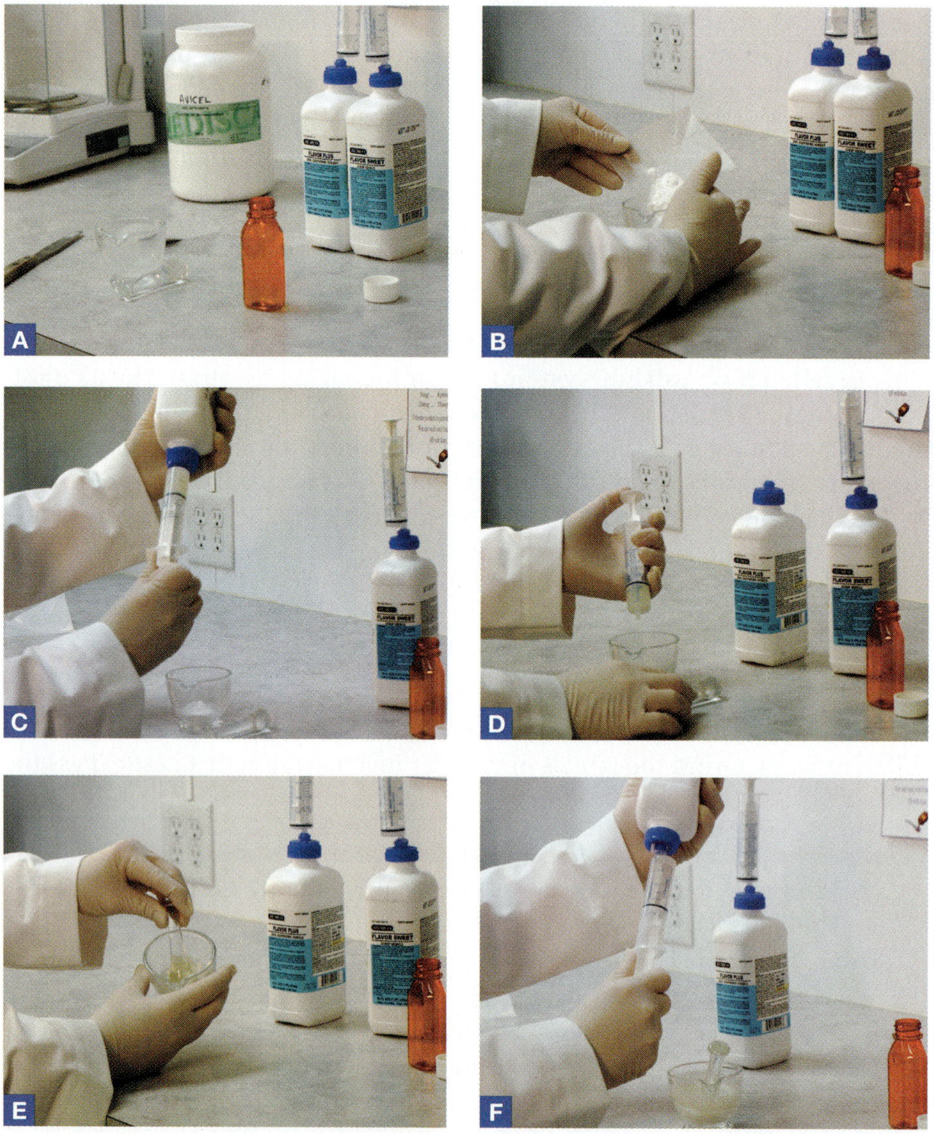

Figure 7-1
Compounding a suspension

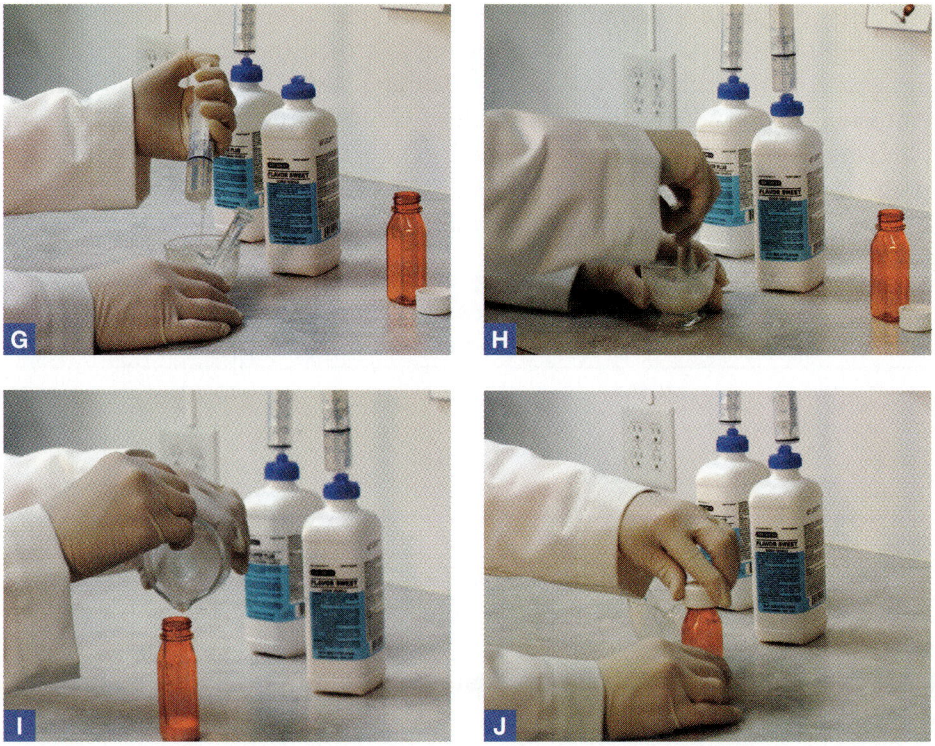

Figure 7-1
Compounding a suspension (*continued*)

EMULSIONS

Emulsions are more complicated to prepare. The components of an emulsion cannot be simply mixed together to form an emulsion. Preparing emulsions requires an energy source that will break up the oil and water liquids and increase the surface area of the internal phase. Several manual and mechanical methods can be used to prepare emulsions: English Method, Continental Method, bottle method, and beaker method. Table 7-6 lists equipment that can be used to prepare emulsions.

TABLE 7-6 Equipment Used to Prepare Emulsions

Equipment	Note(s)
Mortar and Pestle	Mortar should have a rough surface to shear liquid into globules.
Bottle	For shaking—eliminates splashing and loss of product.
Beaker	Requires a hot plate and stirrer.
Mechanical Stirrer or Mixer	Commercially available and can be found in department, gourmet kitchen stores, or a kitchen supplies wholesaler.
Homogenizer	Manual or electric; uses high pressure shearing action.

The English Method is also called the wet gum method. A **mucilage** is prepared by adding a small quantity of water to the gum or hydrocolloid and then triturated or mixed until the mixture is uniform. The oil component is added in small quantities by using rapid **trituration**, resulting in a thick, viscous mixture. More water is slowly added and the mixture is rapidly triturated until the emulsion is formed.

mucilage
sticky mixture

trituration
the act of reducing a drug to a fine powder

The Continental Method is known as the dry gum method. The gum or hydrocolloid is rapidly mixed with the oil, and then the water is added all at once with rapid trituration. When a snapping sound is heard, the primary emulsion has formed. More water is added slowly with rapid trituration until the emulsion has completely formed. The oil:water:emulsifier ratio for preparing the primary emulsion is 4:2:1. The component ratios for preparing the primary emulsions are listed in Table 7-7.

TABLE 7-7 Component Ratios for Compounding Primary Emulsions

Oil	Acacia	Tragacanth
Fixed oils (vegetable oils)	4:2:1	40:20:1
Mineral oil	3:2:1	30:20:1
Linseed oil	2:2:1	20:20:1
Volatile oils	2:2:1	20:20:1

The bottle or shaking method can be used with emulsions that contain volatile oils and is a variation of the dry gum method. The gum and oil are added to the bottle and shaken with a short, rapid movement. The water is added all at once and the mixture is rapidly shaken again to form the primary emulsion. Water can be added in smaller amounts and shaken to form the final emulsion.

The beaker method is used with synthetic emulsifying agents. It involves heating each phase, oil and water, separately to about 60°C to 70°C. The internal phase is stirred into the external phase. The mixture is then removed from the heat and stirred gently and periodically until it is congealed and cooled.

FLAVORING

An oral liquid may be compounded properly, but if the compound does not taste good, the patient may become noncompliant with the treatment. Certain sweeteners (such as saccharin, sucrose, asulfame, stevia, or aspartame) and flavoring agents can be used to mask some basic tastes. See Chapter 10, "Medication Flavoring," for complete information.

Quality Control

All compounding activities should include triple checks on all weights or measurements and documentation of all steps, weight or measurements, calculations, and end-product testing as part of a good quality assurance program. Quality control and end-product testing should include checking the final volume or weight, appearance, odor, and pH of the compounded product. Solutions need to be checked for clarity or particulate matter. Suspensions and emulsions have other characteristics that need to be checked.

Suspensions should be checked for the extent of settling of the undissolved particles. If a batch is prepared of a suspension, all of the bottles in the batch should settle evenly and the height of the settling should be the same for each bottle. The particles should not form a solid "cake" or mass at the bottom of the bottle. Suspensions should also be checked for ease of dispersibility or the ability to resuspend the solid particles in the liquid vehicle by shaking the bottle. Shaking the bottle should easily resuspend the solid particles, and the liquid should look uniform once shaken. Finally, the suspension should be pourable, even after refrigeration. If there is a problem with any of these characteristics, it should be brought to the attention of the pharmacist so that proper adjustments can be made.

Emulsions should be checked for signs of creaming, coalescence, and mold or bacteria growth. Although generally not practical, a microscope can also be used to check globule sizes. Creaming occurs when the globules clump together or flocculate and concentrate in one specific part of an emulsion. The compound looks clumpy and "cottage-cheese-like," and the drug is not evenly distributed in the product. Creaming is easily reversible by simply shaking the compound. On the other hand, coalescence or "cracking" of the emulsion is irreversible. The globules are destroyed in the emulsion, and the oil and water phases are completely separate.

A technician should immediately alert the pharmacist if the compounded solution, suspension, or emulsion does not appear as expected or there are abnormal test results. In either case, the product should not be dispensed. The pharmacist may need to make adjustments in the formulation to correct the problem or perhaps to make the compound more stable.

Packaging

Solutions can generally be packaged in glass or plastic containers. Many drugs can degrade when exposed to light; therefore, the container should be light-resistant or amber-colored. Solutions have many different applications and may be packaged in amber oval bottles, dropper bottles, squeeze bottles, applicator bottles, or spray bottles (Figure 7-2).

Suspensions and emulsions should be packaged in tight containers that have a large opening to allow easy pouring of a viscous or thick liquid. There should be sufficient headspace in the container to allow the compounded suspension or emulsion to be shaken. Suspensions for otic or ophthalmic use should be dispensed in sterile dropper bottles as well. Squeeze bottles can be used for topical liquid emulsions, whereas tubes or containers with a pump dispenser can be used for viscous cream emulsions.

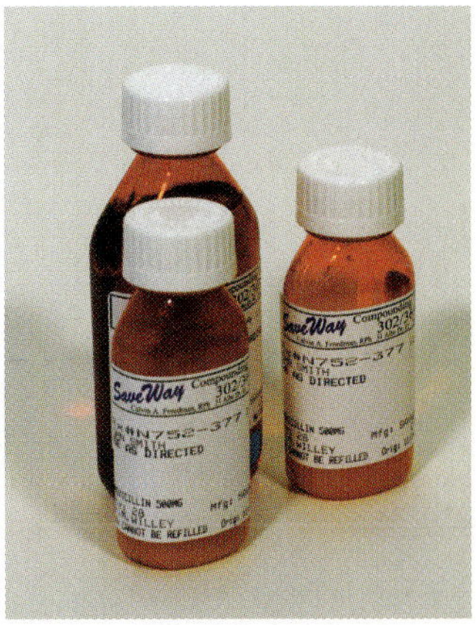

Figure 7-2 Packaged solutions, suspensions, and emulsions

Labeling

The following information should be included on all compounding labels: generic or chemical name of the active ingredient(s), strength or quantity, an assigned pharmacy lot number, beyond-use or expiration dating, storage requirements, and instructions for use. Suspensions and emulsions also require "Shake Well" auxillary labels (Figure 7-3).

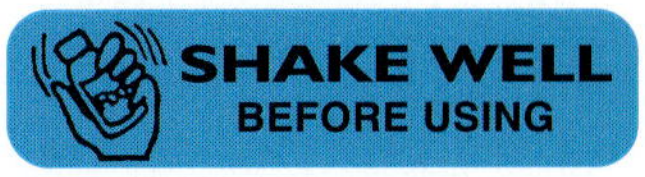

Figure 7-3 Auxiliary label

Stability

If no information is available, beyond-use dates are assigned as described in the section "Stability Criteria and Beyond-Use Dating" in the general test chapter "Pharmaceutical Compounding Nonsterile Preparations (795)."

Extended beyond-use dates may be used if supported by appropriate literature sources, such as published studies in journals, or by direct testing evidence.

Aqueous or water-based compounded liquids should be assigned a 14-day expiration date when stored at cold temperatures. Nonaqueous or oil-based liquids prepared with a manufactured product should be assigned an expiration date of six months or 25 percent of the manufacturer's expiration date, whichever is less. For all other products, a 30-day expiration date or the intended duration of therapy can be assigned, whichever is less.

Fixed oil suspensions are generally more stable than aqueous based solutions and less susceptible to chemical degradation. They may have longer beyond-use expiration dates than solutions. However, if water is present in the suspension, it generally has a short beyond-use date. Suspensions made with approved suspending agents, such as Ora-Plus®, may also have an extended beyond use date. The stability for each compounded suspension, whether in oil or made by using a suspending agent, must be considered individually. In most circumstances where there is a published formula or recipe, the expiration of the product or beyond-use dating will be indicated.

Emulsions are subject to the same beyond-use dating criteria as solutions, since there is an aqueous component. There are factors that can enhance the stability of an emulsion:

- decreasing the globule size of the internal phase
- obtaining an optimum ratio of oil to water
- increasing the viscosity of the emulsion

Patient Counseling

The patient or caregiver should be asked if he would like counseling about the compound from the pharmacist. Since these oral liquids are taken internally and absorbed systemically, there may be side effects that the patient should be made aware of. Prior to dispensing, the patient or caregiver should be instructed on how to store the product. With suspensions and emulsions, the patient or caregiver should also be instructed to shake the bottle well just prior to measuring out the dose to be taken. He should also be instructed to call the pharmacy if the appearance or odor of the liquid has changed in any way. Any change should be suspect, as it may indicate contamination. It is always safest to contact the pharmacist or take the product to a pharmacy.

SUMMARY

While tablets and capsules are the most common dosage forms for medications in general, liquids are the most common dosage form for compounded medications. The variety of routes of administration and patient compliance are just two of the reasons for the number of compounded liquids. While most are relatively simple to compound compared with other dosage forms, many special considerations must be factored, and as always, accuracy and attention to detail are vital.

PROFILES OF PRACTICE

Sample Formula: Oral Suspension

for training purposes only

Lactose	5 g
Ora-Sweet	20 ml
Glycerin USP	to wet
Stevioside 15% Liq. Extract	4 gtts
Flavor	1 ml
Ora-Plus	50 ml

1. Accurately measure each ingredient.
2. In a mortar, wet the lactose with the glycerin until a smacking sound is created.
3. Add Ora-Sweet to mixture and mix well.
4. Add flavor and stevioside to mixture and mix well.
5. Pour mixture into a 2 oz. amber bottle.
6. Add Ora-Plus to the amber bottle and mix well.

Sample Formula: Massage Lotion (Emulsion)

for training purposes only

Safflower oil	30 ml
Glycerin	20 ml
Rose oil	2 ml
Polysorbate 80	2 ml
Benzyl alcohol	1 ml
Purified water	qs

1. Accurately measure each ingredient.
2. Mix both oils and polysorbate 80.
3. Mix the glycerin with the benzyl alcohol, then add 45 ml of purified water to create an aqueous phase.
4. Add the oil mixture to the aqueous phase and mix well.
5. Package and label.

PROFILES OF PRACTICE

CHAPTER TERMS

aromatic waters
clear, saturated aqueous solutions of volatile oils or aromatic substances; may be used internally or externally

buffers
ingredients that prevent change in the concentration of another chemical substance

co-solvent system
two ingredients together used as a solvent

elixirs
solutions that are sweetened and alcohol-based

emulsions
a type of suspension consisting of two immiscible liquids and an emulsifying agent to hold them together

geriatric
referring to a senior patient

hydrophilic
readily absorbing moisture

hydrophobic
property of repelling water

mucilage
sticky mixture

solutions
clear liquid preparations in which all of the ingredients are dissolved in a suitable vehicle; may contain one or more active ingredients

suspensions
liquids that contain ingredients, both active and inert, that are not soluble in the vehicle, but rather suspended or resuspended upon shaking

trituration
the act of reducing a drug to a fine powder

CHAPTER 7

CHAPTER REVIEW QUESTIONS

1. How many different types of solutions are there?
   a. 3
   b. 5
   c. 9
   d. 4

2. Suspensions are considered to be a(n) ____________ system.
   a. emollient forming
   b. thick liquid
   c. two phased
   d. co-solvent

3. Why are preservatives added to a compounded liquid?
   a. to prevent microbial contamination
   b. to help camouflage the taste of bitter medicines
   c. to make the liquid easier to pour
   d. to help keep the color consistent

4. If a mixture is hydrophobic, what can be added to help?
   a. glycerin
   b. magnesium carbonate
   c. alcohol
   d. distilled water

5. Which of the following are standard methods to prepare emulsions?
   a. English Method
   b. Continental Method
   c. Bottle method
   d. all of the above

6. True or false: Ethanol alcohol is the only alcohol that should be used in oral elixirs.
   a. true
   b. false

7. True or false: If no information is available, beyond-use dates are assigned as described in the section "Stability Criteria and Beyond-Use Dating" in the general test chapter "Pharmaceutical Compounding Nonsterile Preparations (795)."
   a. true
   b. false

8. What are the five types of solutions?

9. Define trituration.

10. **Critical Thinking** Name the factors that have to be considered when preparing any oral liquid, and explain why.

Resources and References

1. Allen, Loyd V. Jr., Ph.D. *The Art, Science, and Technology of Pharmaceutical Compounding*. Washington, DC: American Pharmaceutical Association, 1998.
2. "Stability Criteria and Beyond-Use Dating—Pharmaceutical Compounding Nonsterile Preparations." (795) In: *United States Pharmacopeia 27/National Formulary 22*. Rockville, MD: United States Pharmacopeial Convention, 2003.

CHAPTER 8

Ointments, Creams, Pastes, and Gels

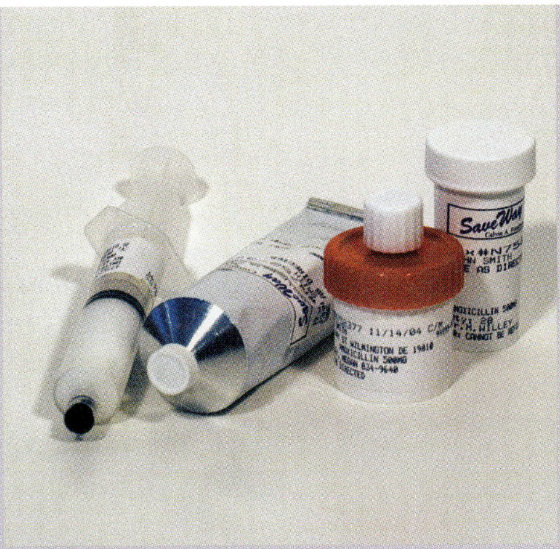

Learning Objectives

After completing this chapter, you should be able to:

- Identify the different types of ointments, creams, pastes, and gels.
- Distinguish the ingredients and composition properties required to prepare ointments, creams, pastes, and gels.
- Explain the procedures and techniques used to prepare ointments, creams, pastes, and gels.
- State how to perform quality control testing of ointments, creams, pastes, and gels.
- Select appropriate packaging for the compounded ointments, creams, pastes, and gels.
- List the labeling requirements for ointments, creams, pastes, and gels.
- Evaluate the stability of ointments, creams, pastes, and gels in assigning beyond-use dates and storage requirements.

INTRODUCTION

Ointments, creams, pastes, and gels are topical, nonsterile, semisolid products that are commonly compounded in pharmacies. They are typically applied to the skin to treat various disorders.

Types and Definitions

Ointments, creams, pastes, and gels have three main functions:

- To protect an injured area from the environment and permit healing
- To hydrate the skin or produce an emollient effect
- To treat or medicate, either locally or systematically, by application to the skin

The drug penetration and effect is dependent on several factors:

- The amount of pressure and rubbing involved in applying the topical product
- The surface area where the topical product is applied
- The skin's condition, healthy and unbroken, or injured or inflamed
- The based used in the topical product
- The use of occlusive dressings

All topical bases are classified according to two different methods: the degree of skin penetration and the relationship of water to the base composition. Table 8-1 summarizes both classification methods.

OINTMENTS

ointment
semi-solid topical preparations that are applied to the skin or mucous membranes

Ointments are semi-solid topical preparations that are applied to the skin or mucous membranes. They soften or melt at body temperature, spread easily, and are nongritty or smooth in texture. There are several types of ointments, including oleaginous bases, absorption bases, water-in-oil or oil-in-water emulsion bases, and water-soluble bases. Table 8-2 summarizes the types of ointments and their characteristics.

PASTES

paste
stiff or very viscous ointments that do not melt or soften at body temperature

Pastes are stiff or very viscous ointments that do not melt or soften at body temperature. They are intended to be used as protectant coverings over the areas where they are applied. Pastes usually contain at least 20 percent solids. An example of a paste is zinc oxide paste 25 percent, USP. This product is used to prevent diaper rash or protect certain body parts, such as the nose, from sunburn.

CREAMS

cream
opaque, soft solids or thick liquids for topical use

Creams are opaque, soft solids or thick liquids for topical use. They are primarily water-in-oil or oil-in-water emulsion bases. The active ingredient(s) is dissolved or suspended in water soluble or vanishing cream bases. Creams are used externally and generally dissipate into the skin upon application.

GELS

gel
semi-solid systems consisting of suspensions made up of small inorganic particles or of large organic molecules interpenetrated by a liquid

Gels are semi-solid systems consisting of suspensions made up of small inorganic particles or of large organic molecules interpenetrated by a liquid. There are two types of classification systems for gels. According to the USP, they can be classified as either inorganic, two-phase systems or organic,

TABLE 8-1 Classification of Topical Bases

Base Type	Skin Penetration	Example Bases
Epidermic[a]	None or very little	Oleaginous
Endothermic[b]	Into the dermis	Absorption
Diadermic[c]	Into and through the skin	Emulsion, water soluble

[a]The external layer of skin.
[b]The internal layer of skin.
[c]Going through the skin.

TABLE 8-2 Summary of Ointment Bases

Base Type	Description	Example
Oleaginous	Water insoluble Not water washable Will not absorb water Emollient Occlusive Greasy	White petrolatum White ointment
Absorption	Water insoluble Not water washable Will absorb water Emollient Occlusive Greasy	Hydrophylic petrolatum *Aquabase®* *Aquaphor®* *Hydrophor®*
W/O Emulsion	Water insoluble Not water washable Will absorb water Contains water Emollient Occlusive Greasy	Cold cream Lanolin, hydrous *Hydrocream®* *Eucerin®* *Nivea®*
O/W Emulsion	Water insoluble Water washable Contains water Nonocclusive Nongreasy	Hydrophylic ointment *Dermabase®* *Velvachol®* *Unibase™*
Water Soluble	Water soluble Water washable Will absorb water Anhydrous or hydrous Nonocclusive Nongreasy	Polyethylene glycol (PEG) ointment

single-phase systems. If the particle size is large in a two-phase system, it is called a **magma**. Single-phase systems consist of organic macromolecules dispersed throughout a liquid phase, but there are no clear separation or boundaries between the macromolecules and the liquid. The macromolecules may be synthetic or may consist of natural gums or mucilages. The usual liquid phase is water, but it can be alcohol or oleaginous. Gels can also be classified as iic hydrogels or organogels. Table 8-3 summarizes the general classifications of gels.

magma
a particle size that is large in a two-phase system

Most gels are absorption bases and have the following characteristics: water washable, water soluble, water absorbing, and greaseless. The gel should have clarity and sparkle and should maintain its viscosity over a wide temperature range.

TABLE 8-3 General Classification of Gels

Class	USP Class	Type	Examples
Hydrogels	Inorganic	Aqueous	Silica, bentonite, pectin, sodium alginate, alumina, methylcellulose
Organogels	Organic	Hydrocarbon	Petrolatum, mineral oil/polyethelene gel, *Plastibase*®
		Animal or vegetable fats	Lard, cocoa butter
		Soap base greases	Aluminum stearate with heavy mineral oil gel
		Hydrophilic polar or nonionic	*Carbowax*® bases (PEG ointment)
Hydrogels	Organic	Organic	Pectin paste, tragacanth jelly Methylcellulose, sodium
	Organic	Natural and synthetic gums	carboxymethylcellulose, *Pluronic F-127*™
	Inorganic	Inorganic	Bentonite gel (10–25%), *Veegum*™

Composition and Ingredients

Ointments, pastes, and creams can include the following components: active ingredient(s), stiffeners, oleaginous components, water components, emulsifying agents, humectants, preservatives, penetration enhancers, and antioxidants. Some components are discussed in detail in the "Preparation and Compounding Techniques" section of this chapter.

Ideally, pure drug from a USP/NF powder is the best source of active ingredients to prepare topical products. If the pure drug cannot be obtained, injectable forms of the drug are a good alternative source because they usually contain very few excipients. If the injectable is premixed, concentration should be considered. Incorporating too much liquid into a topical application can cause it to be too thin, and it may "run off." If the injectable comes with diluent, sometimes you can use a lesser amount to dissolve the drug, making it more concentrated so that a lesser volume is incorporated. Tablets and capsules should be the last resort due to the high excipient content. The excipients in tablets and capsules may cause the preparation to be too thick, may interfere with penetration, may not reduce to a small enough particle size, or may not dissolve. Many times when using tablets or capsules, the final product is not smooth, but rather gritty. This would not be a "pharmaceutically elegant" product to dispense. Each compound must be considered individually and researched in order to choose the best form for the active ingredient.

Stiffeners enhance the viscosity of the preparation; they are generally waxes with high melting points. Table 8-4 lists the common stiffening agents used in topical preparations.

TABLE 8-4 List of Common Stiffening Agents Used in Topical Products

Castor oil, hydrogenated
Cetostearyl alcohol
Cetyl alcohol
Cetyl esters wax
Hard fat
Paraffin
Synthetic paraffin
Stearyl alcohol
Wax, emulsifying
Wax, white
Wax, yellow

Humectants can be added to decrease water loss from the product, especially after application to the skin. Common humectants include glycerin, propylene glycol, or polyethylene glycol (PEG) 300.

humectants
a substance that promotes the retention of moisture

Some products are susceptible to degradation via oxidation or exposure to air. Antioxidants, such as butylated hydroxyl toluene, are added to decrease this type of rancidification.

Penetration or absorption enhancers interact with both the active drug and the outer skin layer (called the stratum corneum) to increase the absorption of the drug through the skin. A gel basically consists of a liquid phase, which can be aqueous, alcoholic, or oleaginous; a gelling agent; and possibly a preservative. Gelling agents increase the viscosity of the liquid base and form the macromolecules. Table 8-5 contains a list of common gelling agents used.

Preparation and Compounding Techniques

Quite often, topical preparations are compounded by simply combining two or more commercial products together. With these compounds, it is important to remember to combine "like" products, such as cream with cream or ointment with ointment. Mixing a cream and an ointment together can sometimes lead to incompatibilities, and the two components will separate. Occasionally,

TABLE 8-5 List of Gelling Agents

Acacia	Guar gum	Povidone
Alginic acid	Hydroxyethylcellulose	Propylene carbonate
Bentonite	Hydroxypropyl cellulose	Propylene glycol alginate
Carbomer	Hydroxypropyl methylcellulose	Sodium alginate
CMC sodium	Magnesium aluminum silicate	Sodium starch glycolate
Cetostearyl alcohol	Maltodextrin	Starch
Colloidal silicon dioxide	Methylcellulose	Tragacanth
Ethylcellulose	Polyvinyl alcohol (PVA)	Xantham gum
Gelatin		

ointments, creams, and pastes are compounded from separate components. Gels are more commonly prepared from separate components.

There are basically two methods used to compound topical products: manual and mechanical. Manual methods primarily use a pill or ointment tile and spatula, or a mortar and pestle, to mix the ingredients of the topical product together (Figure 8-1 A-I). The advantages of using an ointment tile are as follows:

Figure 8-1
Compounding with an ointment tile

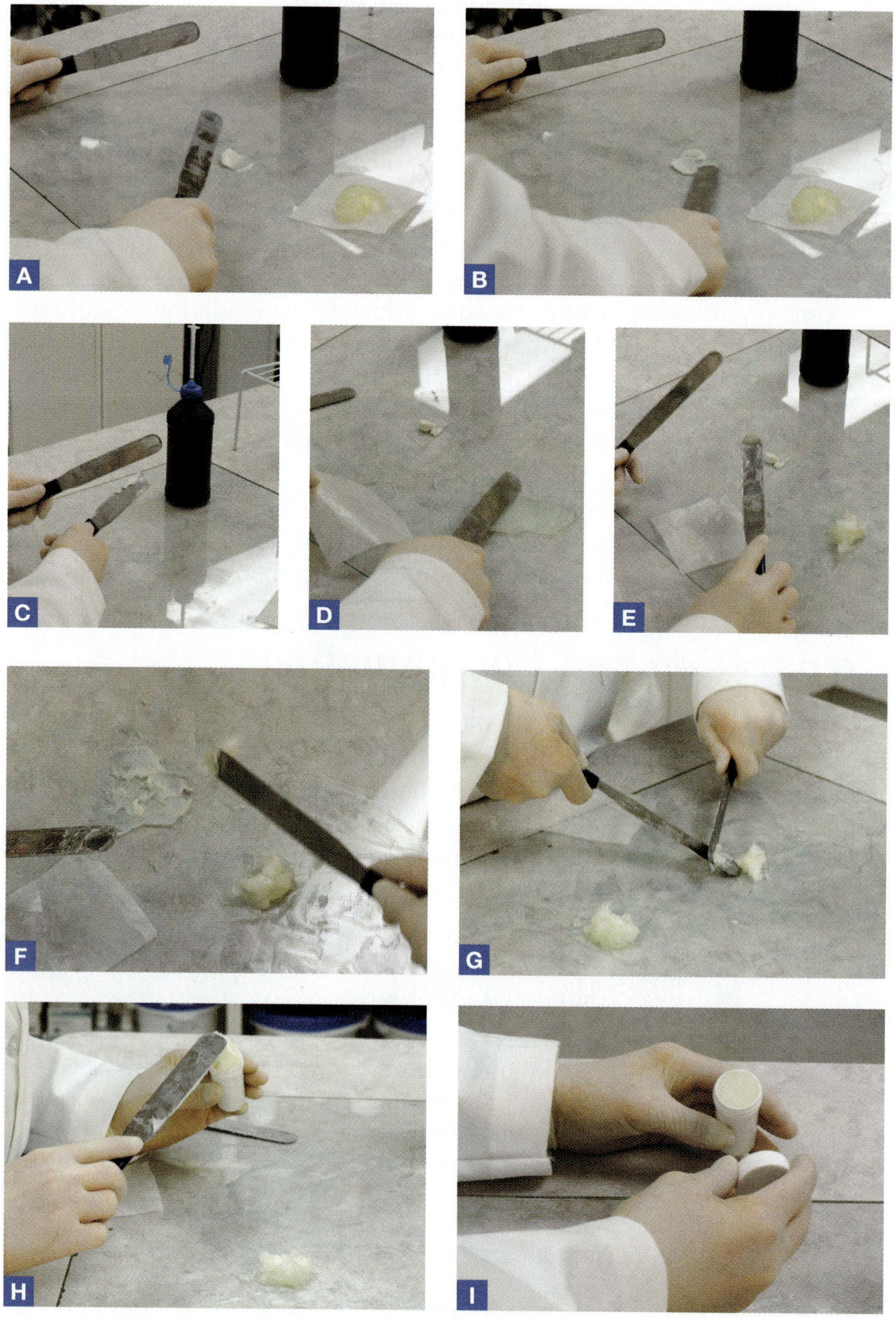

- It can be used to reduce the particle size of powders.
- The ointment can be thoroughly mixed on the tile.
- The tile can be easily cleaned after use.

The "bag" method (Figure 8-2 A-H) is another manual method to mix ointments, creams, or gels. The ingredients (active drugs and base) may be sealed into a zip-lock bag. The contents are kneaded together by squeezing the bag until a uniform mixture is obtained.

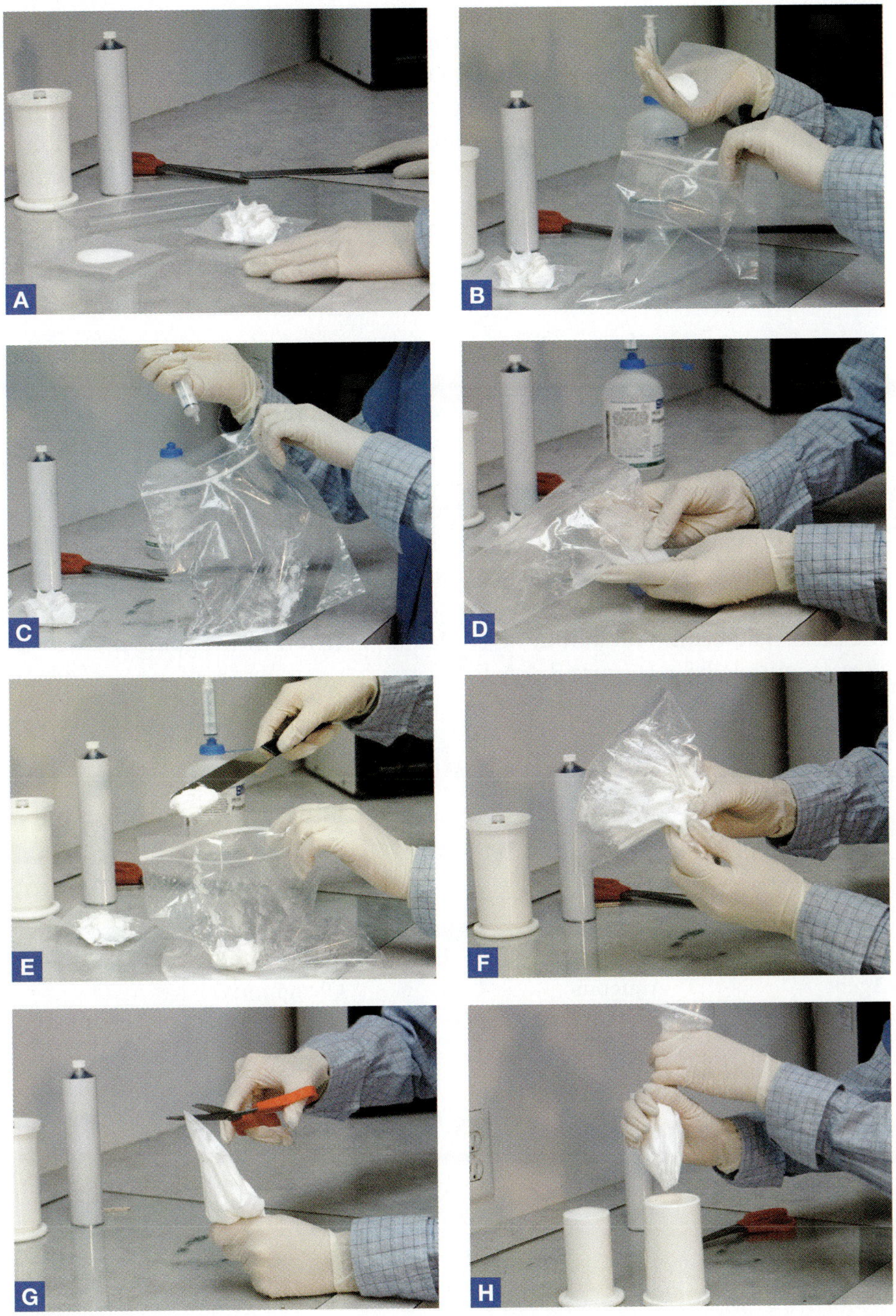

Figure 8-2
Compounding using the "bag" method

WORKPLACE WISDOM

When using the bag method, a corner of the bag can be snipped off with scissors and the final product can be squeezed into the final container, similar to the procedure that bakers use to prepare frosting and decorate cakes.

If large quantities of topical products are being compounded, mechanical methods may be the best option. It is wise to invest in a commercial mixer, such as a professional Kitchen-Aid® mixer with large mixing or dough paddles. Ointment mills are also useful in reducing particle size, providing high shear to create micelles needed to prepare PLO gels, and thoroughly mixing the batch.

OLEAGINOUS BASES

After accurately weighing or measuring each ingredient, pulverize the dry ingredients into a fine powder. **Levigate** the powder with a small amount of the base. This can be achieved by mixing the powder with a levigating agent and mixing it with the ointment base on the ointment tile (see Table 8-6). The remainder of the base is added by geometric dilution. (Geometric dilution is the process of mixing a portion of the powder mixture with equal parts of the oleaginous base and repeating until the entire amounts are mixed.) (Figure 8-3 A-H)

levigate
to make smooth

WORKPLACE WISDOM

Another method is to melt a small portion of the base and mix the powder into the melted base until it is dissolved or a uniform mixture is achieved. If the base is melted, it should be stirred occasionally and allowed to cool slowly to prevent the product from becoming lumpy.

ABSORPTION BASES

Absorption bases are formed by adding a w/o emulsion to an oleaginous base. There are several commercial bases available. Emulsifying agents and preservatives may be necessary to obtain a stable final product.

To incorporate water soluble ingredients into the ointment, dissolve the water soluble ingredient in a small amount of water. Use levigation and geometric dilution to mix the aqueous solution in the absorption base. Alternatively, the base may be melted and the solution may be added and stirred into the base. The ointment should be cooled and stirred in the same manner as the oleaginous base (Figure 8-4 A-F).

WATER-IN-OIL EMULSION BASES

Water-in-oil emulsion bases are prepared by adding water to an absorption base. There are several commercial bases available.

TABLE 8-6 List of Levigating Agents Used to Prepare Ointments

Agent	Aqueous Systems	O/W Dispersions	Oleaginous Systems	W/O Dispersions
Castor Oil			X	X
Cottonseed Oil			X	X
Glycerin	X	X		
Mineral Oil, heavy			X	X
Mineral Oil, light			X	X
PEG 400	X	X		
Propylene glycol	X	X		
Tween 80			X	X

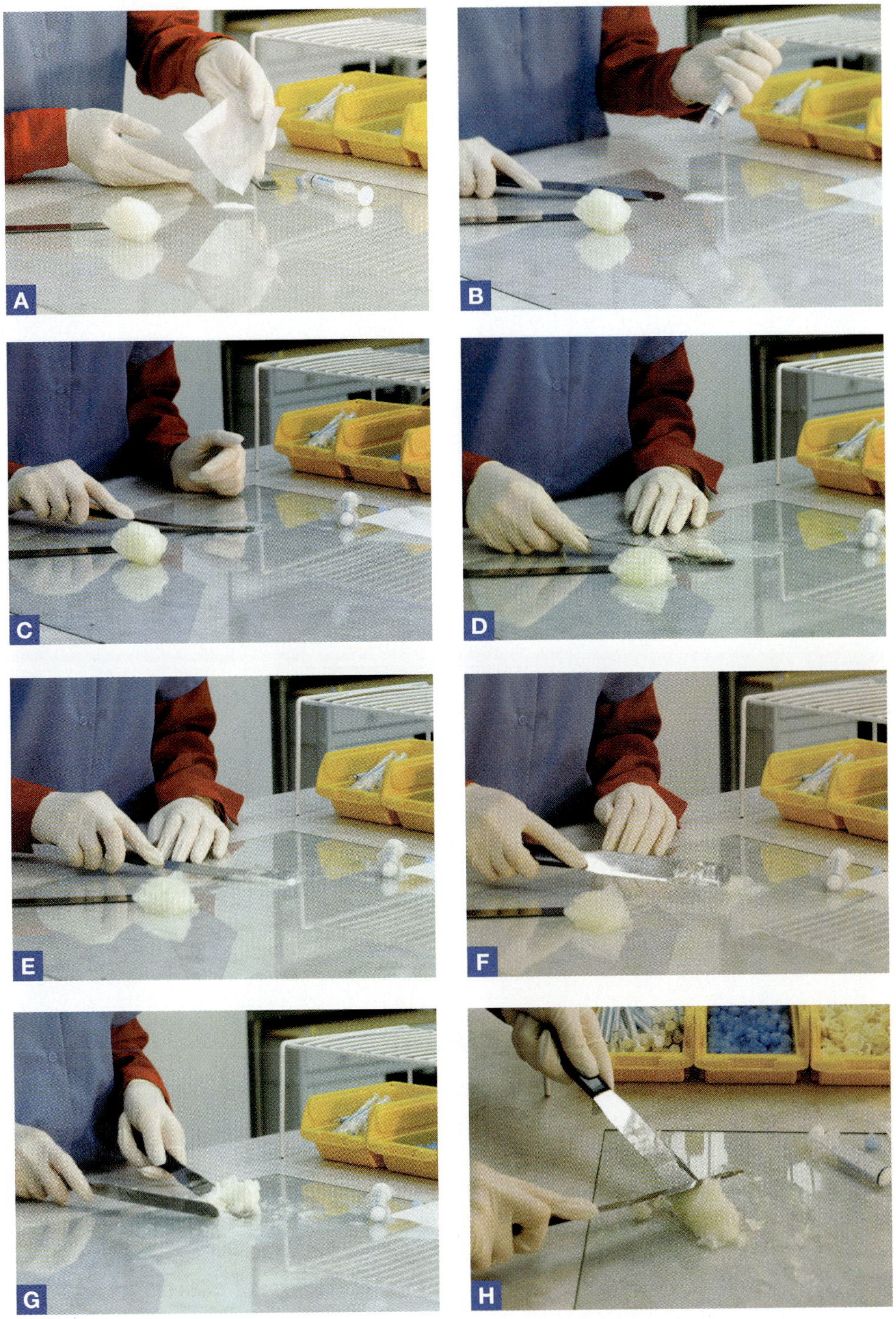

Figure 8-3
Compounding with an oleaginous base

Incorporate the oil or powder into the base by using an ointment tile or mortar and pestle. If a large quantity of powder needs to be added, a levigating agent may be used. The levigated mixture is mixed in the w/o emulsion base. Alternatively, the base may be melted and the levigated mixture may be added and mixed into the base. Heat should be kept to a minimum amount of time to prevent water loss and an increase in viscosity of the final product.

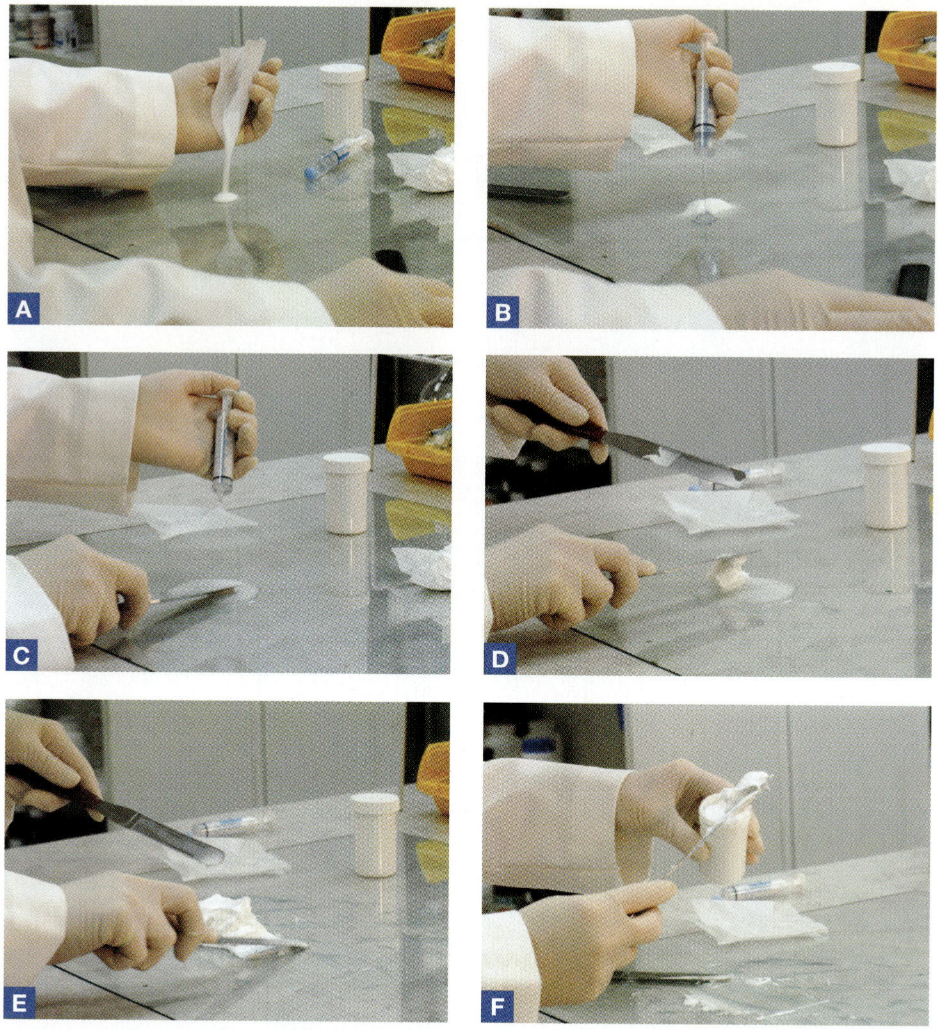

Figure 8-4
Compounding with an absorption base

OIL-IN-WATER EMULSION BASES

Oil-in-water emulsion bases are also known as vanishing creams because they disappear or vanish upon application to the skin. There are several commercial products available.

The powder may be dissolved in a small amount of water to form an aqueous solution and then be added to the o/w emulsion base, using the same manual method as the absorption base. A small amount of oil may be incorporated into the base, as there is usually an excess of emulsifying agent. If a large amount of oil needs to be added, a small amount of o/w surfactant may be added to assist in uniformly dispersing the oil in the base. Again, if heat is used, it should be kept to a minimum to prevent water loss and the development of a stiff and waxy final product.

WATER SOLUBLE BASES

Water-soluble ingredients may be dissolved in a small amount of water before incorporating them into the base by using an ointment tile or mortar and pestle.

Insoluble powders can be levigated with a small quantity of PEG 400, glycerin, or propylene glycol and incorporated into the base by using an ointment tile or mortar and pestle. Oils may need to be in a solvent such as glycerin or propylene glycol prior to mixing them in the water-soluble base to enhance the stability of the final product. If large amounts of water or aqueous solutions need to be added, it may be necessary to heat the base in a water bath to mix and prepare the final product (Figure 8-5 A-I).

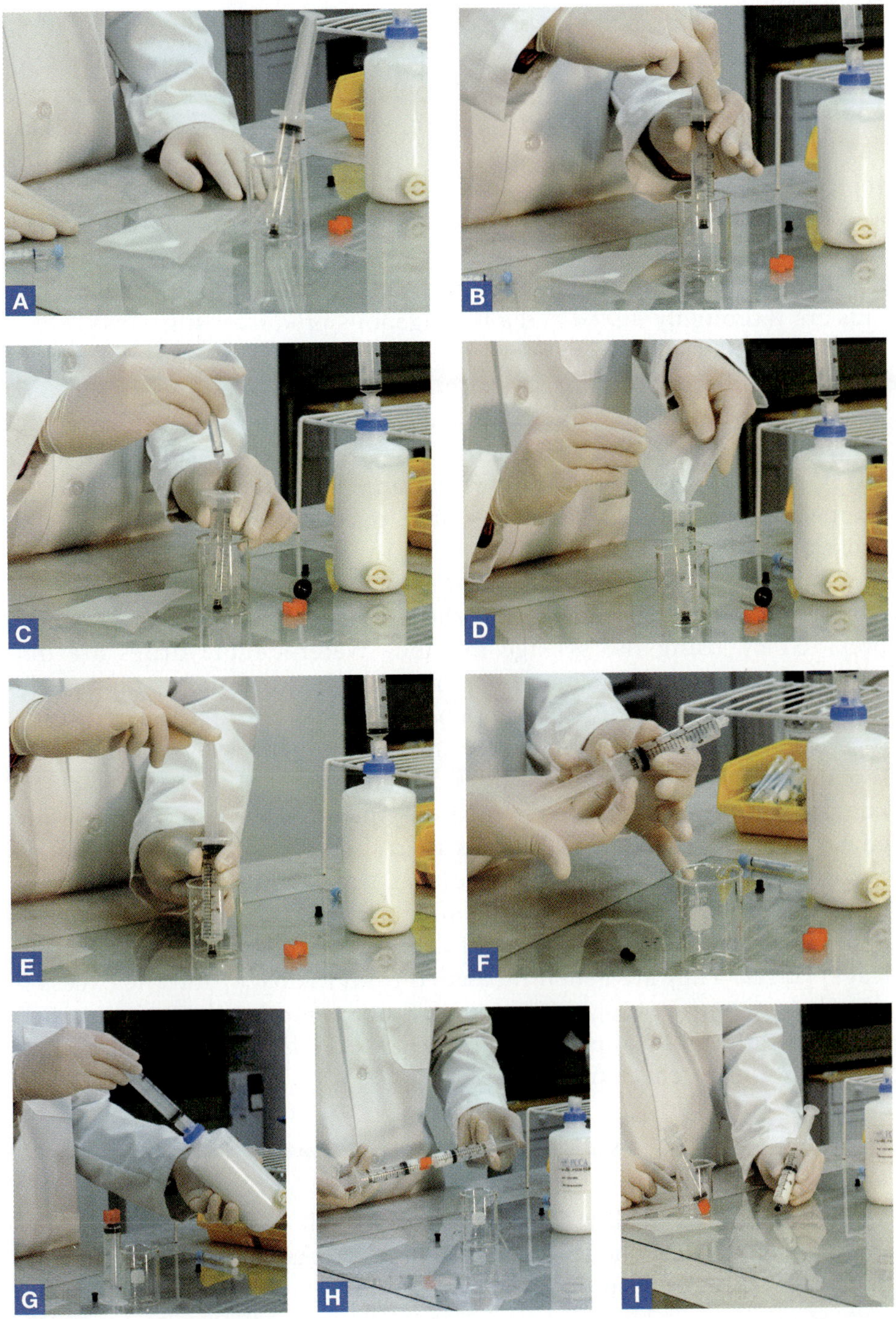

Figure 8-5
Compounding with a water soluble base

GELS

The preparation method for a gel is dependent on the gelling agent. Most gels are prepared by dissolving the gelling agent in a water base, although alcohol or oil may also be used. Each gelling agent is different, and the instruction on the compounding worksheet should be followed carefully. The active ingredient(s) may be added before or after the gel is formed; however, it is best to add it before the gel is formed if the active ingredients do not interfere with the gel formation.

Mixers can be used to prepare gels. The propeller should be kept at the bottom of the container when mixing, and formation of the vortex dissolved, to minimize the incorporation of air bubbles.

Another technique used to prepare gels is the syringe method. This can be done using either two luer-lock syringes, two topical syringes, or a topical syringe and a luer-lock syringe. Ingredients are placed in a syringe, and the air is expelled. The syringe is then attached to another syringe with a connector designed to fit the type(s) of syringe used. The contents are then forced back and forth between the two syringes until the ingredients are thoroughly mixed and a homogenous product results.

PLO gels
Pluronic-lecithin organogels

micelle
a large water drop surrounded by an oil formation

Pluronic-lecithin organogels, or **PLO gels**, have a pluronic component, which is aqueous, and a lecithin component, which is an oil base. When the two components are mixed together, using a high-shear force, it forms a greasy gel containing **micelles**, which are basically large water drops surrounded by an oil formation. The water-soluble drug is trapped in the micelle. PLO gels have excellent skin penetration because the oil layer of the micelle is easily absorbed through the outer layer of skin. Once the micelle is absorbed through the skin, the water component with the drug in absorbed into the body. PLO gels can be prepared by using the syringe method. Water-soluble drugs are dissolved in the pluronic component and drawn up into a syringe. The pluronic component must be kept cold to remain fluid, because it solidifies at room temperature. The lecithin component is drawn up into a separate syringe. The two syringes are connected with a luer lock-to-luer lock connector. The pluronic component is added to the lecithin component syringe. The mixture is then forced back into the other syringe. This process is repeated several times until a uniform gel is formed. The syringes are then disconnected, and the final PLO gel product is added to the final container. PLOs are often dispensed in 1 ml topical syringes. They are generally loaded from the back, and the excess is expelled when the plunger is inserted. Since topical syringes have a hub that generally holds approximately 0.2 ml, the formula should be prepared for 10 percent extra.

Quality Control

As part of a good quality assurance program, all compounding activities should include triple-checks on all weights and measurements, documentation of all steps, weights or measurements used, calculations, and end-product testing. The final product should also be checked for the final weight, visual appearance, color, odor, viscosity, pH, homogenicity or phase separation, particle size uniformity and distribution, and texture.

Packaging

Ointments are primarily packaged in jars or tubes. Pastes, because of their viscosity, are primarily packaged in jars. Creams and gels can be packaged in tubes, jars, pump dispensers, topical syringes, and applicators. Some gels can also be packaged in squeeze bottles. All products, especially gels, should be packaged in air-tight containers to prevent water loss or gain. Carbomer gel products should be packaged in glass, plastic, or resin-lined containers. Aluminum tubes should be used only when a product has a pH less than 6.5. Other metallic materials can be used with products that are a pH of 7.7 or greater (Figure 8-6).

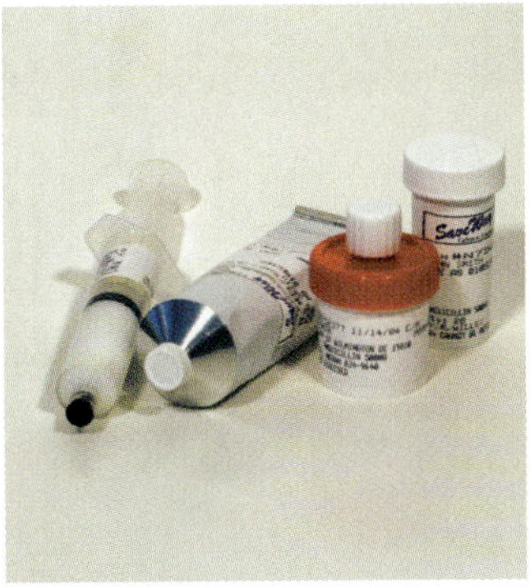

Figure 8-6 Packaged ointments, creams, pastes, and gels

Labeling

The following information should be included on all compounding labels: generic or chemical name of the active ingredient(s), strength and/or quantity, an assigned pharmacy lot number, beyond-use or expiration dating, storage requirements, and instructions for use.

All topical compounded products should be labeled with an "External Use Only" auxiliary label to remind the patient or caregiver that these products are not to be taken orally. Some products may also require a "Refrigerate" auxiliary label (Figure 8-7).

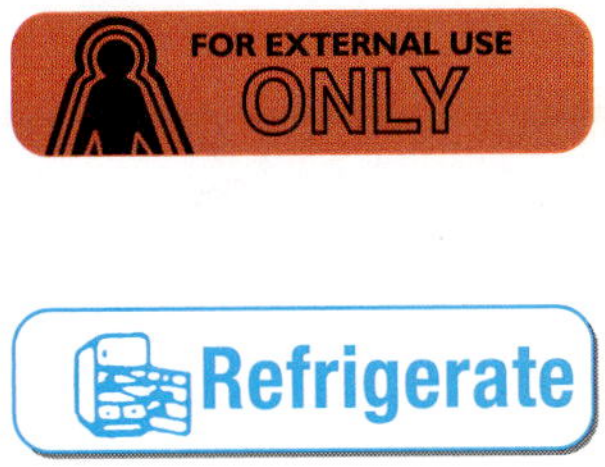

Figure 8-7 Auxiliary labels

Stability

Ointments and pastes are very stable, especially if they are in a fat or oleaginous, anhydrous absorption or anhydrous, water-soluble base. Creams and gels generally contain water and tend to be less stable. However, when preservatives are added or preserved water is used in the formula, the beyond-use date may be extended. This information is usually referenced on the published formula or may be found through research.

If no information is available, beyond-use dates are assigned as described in the section "Stability Criteria and Beyond-Use Dating" in the general test chapter "Pharmaceutical Compounding Nonsterile Preparations (795)." Extended beyond-use dates may be used if supported by appropriate literature sources, such as published studies in journals, or by direct testing evidence.

Aqueous or water-based compounded gels or creams should be assigned a 14-day expiration date when stored at cold temperatures. Nonaqueous or oil-based ointments or pastes prepared with manufactured products should be assigned an expiration date of six months or 25 percent of the manufacturer's expiration date, whichever is shorter. For all other products, a 30-day expiration date or the intended duration of therapy can be assigned, whichever is shorter.

Patient Counseling

The patient or caregiver should be asked if he would like counseling about the compound from the pharmacist. Counseling for topical compounded products may vary depending on the dosage form, active ingredients, and therapeutic outcomes. Generally, only a thin film of an ointment or cream is necessary for treatment. It is applied to the affected area and gently rubbed into the area, unless otherwise instructed. The patient or caregiver should be instructed not to wash the area for at least a couple of hours to allow for proper absorption of the drug and for the drug to be efficacious.

Pastes are viscous and stiff and do not need to be rubbed into the area. They are generally used for a protectant effect and should not be removed until indicated. An example of a paste is zinc oxide paste. It is commonly used to prevent diaper rash because it protects the baby's skin from the harmful effects of urine.

Creams are generally oil-in-water emulsions and can be easily removed with warm water. Aqueous-based gels are also easily removed with water. Ointments and pastes are usually "greasy" and will require warm water, soap, and scrubbing to remove. A protective pad should be recommended if the patient's clothing may come in contact with the topical product.

Prior to dispensing, the patient or caregiver should be instructed on how to store the product. Ointments, creams, and pastes should be stored at room temperature, out of the reach of children, and away from heat and direct sunlight. The patient or caregiver should be instructed to keep gels in tightly closed containers.

SUMMARY

Ointments, creams, pastes, and gels are vehicles used commonly by compounding pharmacies to meet the individual needs of specific patients. There are a number of considerations that must be taken into account (e.g., solubility) when compounding any one of these dosage forms, and the technique used in preparation becomes a true form of art with experience.

PROFILES OF PRACTICE

Sample Formula: Cold Cream

for training purposes only

Cetyl esters wax	25 g
White wax	120 g
Mineral oil	560 g
Sodium borate	5 g
Purified water	qs

1. Accurately measure each ingredient.
2. Break the wax into small pieces, and melt them by using a water bath.
3. Add the mineral oil to the waxes and heat to 70°C.
4. Dissolve the sodium borate in purified water, which has also been heated to 70°C. (Use some of the water from the bath.)
5. Add the dissolved sodium borate to the oleaginous mixture.
6. Remove from heat and stir rapidly.
7. Package and label.

Sample Formula: Carbomer in Alcohol Gel

for training purposes only

70% Isopropyl Alcohol	321.4 ml
Purified Water	125 ml
Carbopol 940	2.25 g
Trolamine NF	3 ml

1. Accurately measure each ingredient
2. Mix the purified water and trolamine in a beaker.
3. Mix the alcohol and carbopol in a separate beaker.
4. Combine both mixtures.
5. Package and label.

PROFILES OF PRACTICE

CHAPTER TERMS

cream
opaque, soft solids or thick liquids for topical use

gel
semi-solid systems consisting of suspensions made up of small inorganic particles or of large organic molecules interpenetrated by a liquid

humectants
a substance that promotes the retention of moisture

levigate
to make smooth

magma
a particle size that is large in a two-phase system

micelle
a large water drop surrounded by an oil formation

ointment
semi-solid topical preparations that are applied to the skin or mucous membranes

paste
stiff or very viscous ointments that do not melt or soften at body temperature

PLO gels
Pluronic-lecithin organogels

CHAPTER 8

CHAPTER REVIEW QUESTIONS

1. Pastes usually contain what percentage of solid?
   a. 22% c. 20%
   b. 25% d. 50%

2. What is the purpose of stiffeners in compounding?
   a. enhance the viscosity of the preparation
   b. to give a waxy/shiny appearance to the final product
   c. to hold together the ingredients
   d. to serve as fillers

3. Products (generally waxes) with a high melting point are known as
   a. buffers c. stiffeners
   b. suppositories d. PEGs

4. What is the process that makes a product smooth?
   a. mitigation c. levigation
   b. trituration d. waxing

5. Insoluble powders can be levigated with a small quantity of
   a. PEG 400 c. propylene glycol
   b. glycerin d. all of the above

6. True or false: Because a compound was carefully prepared for the patient and was triple-checked by the pharmacy staff, it is not necessary to counsel the patient when dispensing the compound.
   a. true b. false

7. True or false: A micelle is a large water drop surrounded by an oil formation.
   a. true b. false

8. A PLO gel consists of both water and oil based ingredients. So how does it penetrate the skin?

9. All topical bases are classified according to two different methods. What are they?

10. **Critical Thinking** Describe the "bag" method as it is used in compounding.

Resources and References

1. Allen, Loyd V. Jr., Ph.D. *The Art, Science, and Technology of Pharmaceutical Compounding*. Washington, DC: American Pharmaceutical Association, 1998.
2. Pharmacy Compounding (795) In: *United States Pharmacopeia 25/National Formulary 20*. Rockville, MD: United States Pharmacopeial Convention, 2001.
3. Stability Criteria and Beyond-Use Dating—Pharmaceutical Compounding Nonsterile Preparations (795) In: *United States Pharmacopeia 27/National Formulary 22*. Rockville, MD: United States Pharmacopeial Convention, 2003.

CHAPTER 9

Ophthalmic, Otic, and Nasal Preparations

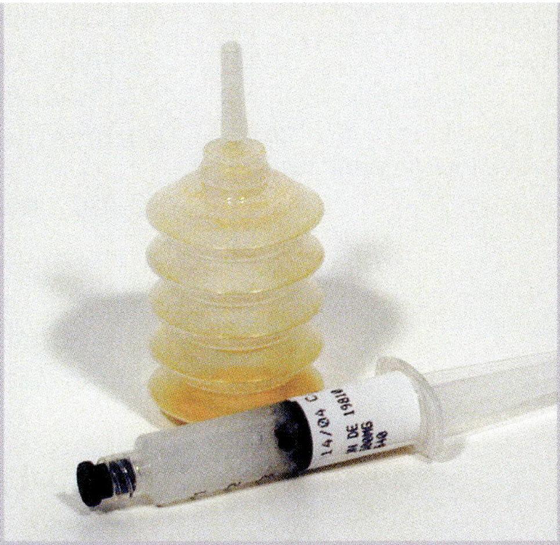

Learning Objectives

After completing this chapter, you should be able to:

- Identify the different types of ophthalmic, otic, and nasal preparations.
- Distinguish the ingredients and composition properties required to prepare ophthalmic, otic, and nasal preparations.
- Describe the procedures and techniques used to compound ophthalmic, otic, and nasal preparations.
- Specify procedures to perform quality control testing on the ophthalmic, otic, and nasal preparations.
- Select appropriate packaging for the compounded ophthalmic, otic, and nasal products.
- Define the labeling requirements for ophthalmic, otic, and nasal preparations.
- Evaluate the stability of ophthalmic, otic, and nasal preparations in assigning beyond-use dates and storage requirements.

INTRODUCTION

Most topical products are prepared in a nonsterile, but clean, environment. However, three types of topical preparations must be prepared as sterile products following the USP 797 standards: ophthalmic products, otic products, and nasal products. This chapter is divided into three major sections, according to the route of administration.

Ophthalmic Dosage Forms

There are three types of ophthalmic dosage forms-solutions, suspensions, and ointments.

TYPES AND DEFINITIONS

Solutions

Ophthalmic solutions are sterile, clear (or particulate-free) liquids intended for instillation in the eye. A solution is the most common ophthalmic dosage form prepared in a compounding pharmacy setting.

Suspensions

Ophthalmic suspensions are sterile liquids that contain solid drug particles in a liquid or other vehicle that is appropriate for the eye. The solid particles have been processed and reduced in

filtration
the passage of a liquid through a filter to sterilize or remove foreign particles

size so that they cannot scratch or irritate the cornea of the eye. Since ophthalmic suspensions must be sterilized by means other than **filtration**, only compounding pharmacies that have the proper sterilization equipment should prepare these products.

Ointments

Ophthalmic ointments are sterile, solid, or semi-solid products that are in a nonaqueous base, such as white petrolatum. The products may or may not contain active drug. Again, these products need to be sterilized by methods other than filtration and must be prepared only in a setting with the proper equipment.

COMPOSITION AND INGREDIENTS

In addition to active drug, ophthalmic preparations require several different ingredients or excipients to make them nonirritating and compatible in the eye. The eye generally tolerates products within a pH range of 4 to 8. Buffers are used in ophthalmic preparations to maintain the pH of the product within the desired range during storage and administration to the eye:

- To maximize comfort for the patient (i.e., little or no stinging)
- To maintain drug stability (i.e., no loss of drug)
- To prevent damage to the eye

Preservatives are necessary when the ophthalmic preparation is intended for multi-use. Preservatives prevent contamination of the preparation due to microbial growth. The pharmacist must make sure that the preservative(s) is compatible with the active drug or other ingredients before adding it to the compound. If the preparation is intended for single use, a preservative may not be necessary. Patients may also have allergies or sensitivities to certain preservatives, and it may be necessary to prepare ophthalmics for these patients without a preservative. This may reduce the length of time the medication is stable and may result in the prescription being refilled more frequently. Table 9-1 lists preservatives commonly used in ophthalmics preparations.

TABLE 9-1 Preservatives Commonly Used in Ophthalmic, Otic, and Nasal Preparations

Preservative	Concentration Range (%)
Chlorobutanol	0.5
Quaternary Ammonium Compounds	0.004–0.02
Benzalkonium chloride	0.013
Bezethonium chloride	0.01
Organic Mercurials	0.001–0.01
Phenylmercuric acetate	0.004
Phenylmercuric nitrate	0.004
Thimerosal	0.01
Parahydroxybenzoates	0.1

TABLE 9-2 Antioxidants Used for Ophthalmic and Nasal Preparations	
Antioxidant	**Usual Maximum Concentration (%)**
Ethylene diamineetraacetic acid	0.1
Sodium bisulfite	0.1
Sodium metabisulfite	0.1
Thiourea	0.1

Some active ingredients in ophthalmics degrade more quickly when exposed to oxygen. Antioxidants may be added to ophthalmics to help stabilize these active ingredients. Table 9-2 lists the antioxidants that may be used.

It is natural for the eye to produce tears that wash foreign substances out of the eye. Tears will also dilute foreign liquids that are instilled in the eye. If an ophthalmic preparation is very "watery," it is almost immediately diluted and washed out by the tears. **Viscosity** enhancers are added to ophthalmic products to make them more viscous or thicker. Increasing the viscosity will increase the time that the ophthalmic preparation remains in the eye. The longer time allows for better drug absorption and effect. Table 9-3 is a list of viscosity enhancers used in ophthalmic products.

viscosity
a physical property of fluids that determines the internal resistance to shear forces

Most ophthalmic solutions are sterilized by passing them through a 0.2 micron filter. Ophthalmic solutions must be free from foreign particles. Filtering the solution will remove these particles to make the solution clear. Wetting or clarifying agents may also be added to achieve clarity. Table 9-4 lists wetting or clarifying agents used in ophthalmic products.

tonicity
a state of normal tension of the tissues by virtue of which the parts are kept in shape, alert, and ready to function in response to a suitable stimulus

Tonicity agents are used to increase comfort when instilling ophthalmic preparations in the eye and to prevent corneal edema or dehydration of the corneal epithelium. Tears are isotonic and equivalent to a 0.9 percent sodium

TABLE 9-3 Viscosity Enhancers Used in Ophthalmic Products	
Viscosity Enhancer	**Usual Concentration (%)**
Hydroxyethylcellulose	0.8
Hydroxypropyl methylcellulose	1
Methylcellulose	2
Polyvinyl alcohol	1.4

TABLE 9-4 Wetting and Clarifying Agents Used in Ophthalmic Preparations	
Agent	**Usual Concentration (%)**
Polysorbate 20	1
Polysorbate 80	1

TABLE 9-5 Tonicity Agents Used in Ophthalmic Preparations		
Agent	NaCl Equivalent (e–1%)	ISO-Osmotic Concentration (%)
Boric Acid	0.52	
Dextrose	0.16	5.51
Glycerin	—	2.6
Mannitol	—	—
Potassium Chloride	0.76	1.19
Sodium Chloride	1	0.9

chloride solution, commonly known as normal saline. Ophthalmic preparations, however, do not necessarily have to be isotonic; it all depends on the preparation's contact with the eye. The eye can tolerate 0.6 to 1.8 percent sodium chloride equivalency. Tonicity is also measured in milliOsmoles per liter (mOsm/L) and can be calculated by the pharmacist. The ideal tonicity value for ophthalmic preparations is 300 mOsm/L; however, a range of 200 to 600 mOsm/L is acceptable.

Some solutions may be hypotonic and need to be adjusted to achieve the proper tonicity range. Table 9-5 lists tonicity agents that are commonly used.

Some solutions may be hypertonic due to the sodium chloride equivalency of the active ingredient(s). Most formulas will contain instructions for adjustment of these ingredients. The pharmacist will determine and calculate which ingredients to adjust in the ophthalmic preparation to achieve the proper tonicity range. This is usually done either by adding a tonicity agent to a hypotonic preparation or by diluting a hypertonic preparation.

PREPARATION AND COMPOUNDING TECHNIQUES

Since ophthalmic preparations are sterile compounds, all compounding personnel—pharmacists and technicians—must be properly trained and validated according to the USP 797 standards prior to compounding them. All compounding must be done in a clean air environment that is at least an ISO Class 8 or Class 100,000. The final sterile preparation is done in a laminar airflow workbench (LAFW) (Figure 9-1) or a barrier isolator, which are ISO Class 5 or Class 100 environments. All of the ingredients used should be of the highest grade that is obtainable and preferably sterile, if possible. Commercially available sterile powders or solutions for parenteral injection may be used.

Ophthalmic solutions may be sterilized by running or pushing the solution through a 0.45 or 0.2 micron sterile membrane filter (Figure 9-2) into a sterile container. Ophthalmic suspensions cannot be sterilized via filtration because the active ingredient(s) would be removed by the filter. Some suspensions and ointments may be **autoclaved** (Figure 9-3). Another sterilization alternative for suspensions or ointments is to sterilize each ingredient in the preparation prior to compounding them together. Dry heat sterilization (Figure 9-4) may be used for dry powders or oils. Aqueous liquids may be

autoclaved
a method of sterilization where heat is used

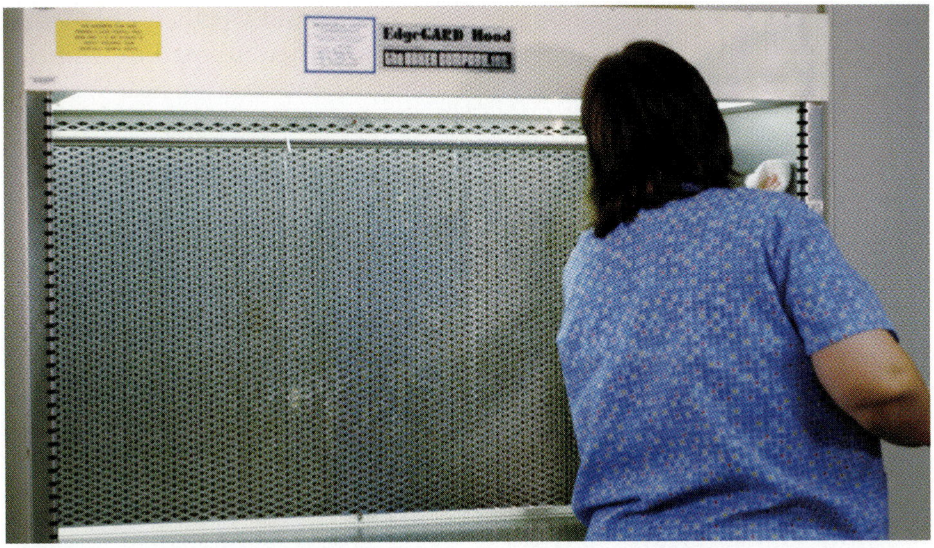

Figure 9-1 LAFW

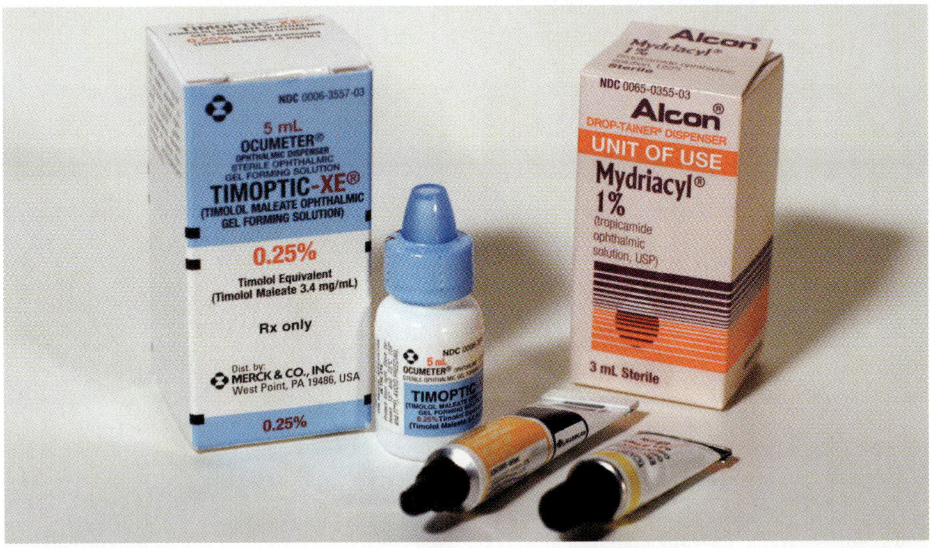

Figure 9-2 Ophthalmic products

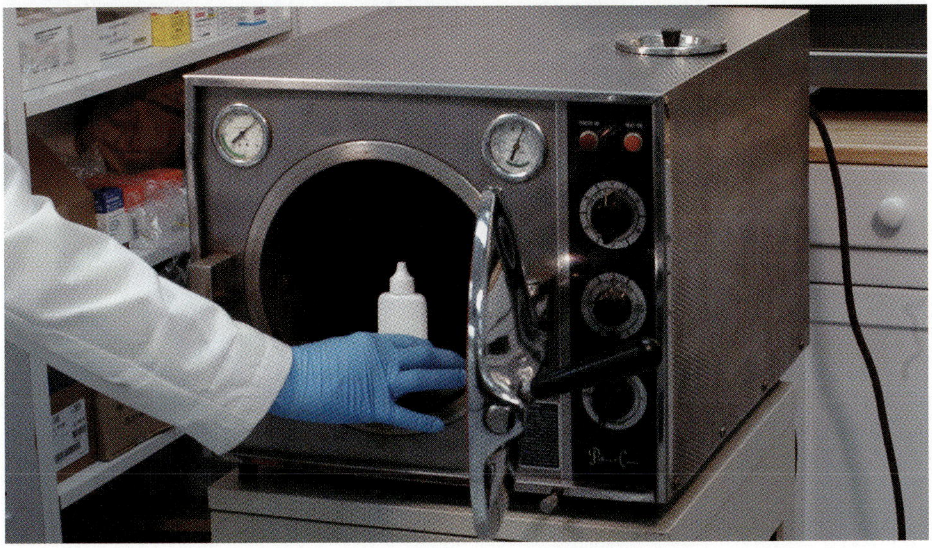

Figure 9-3 Suspensions being autoclaved

WORKPLACE WISDOM

If you ever have a question regarding a compounding procedure—STOP, and check with the pharmacist in charge.

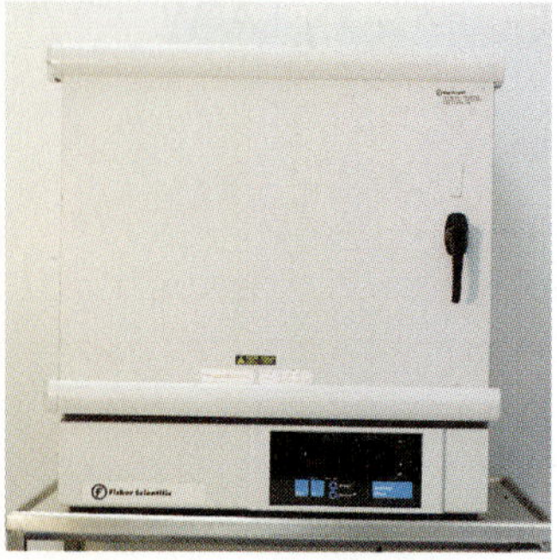

Figure 9-4 Dry heat sterilization

steam autoclaved. It is important to know beforehand whether a particular ingredient is heat labile, meaning it will degrade when exposed to temperatures of a certain degree or higher. Certain ingredients that are heat-sensitive may be gas-sterilized with ethylene oxide.

The sections that follow are the basic step-by-step procedures for compounding each type of ophthalmic preparation. Procedures may vary, depending on the particular compound or pharmacy practice setting.

Solutions

Dissolve the ingredients in about three-fourths of the total quantity of sterile water for injection, or a suitable diluent, and mix well. Add sufficient (QSAD) sterile water or diluent to the desired volume and mix well. Under an LAFW or barrier isolator, using aseptic technique, filter the solution through a sterile 0.2 micron filter into a sterile ophthalmic container. Using a sterile needle and syringe, remove a sample of the solution for quality control testing (Figure 9-5 A-G).

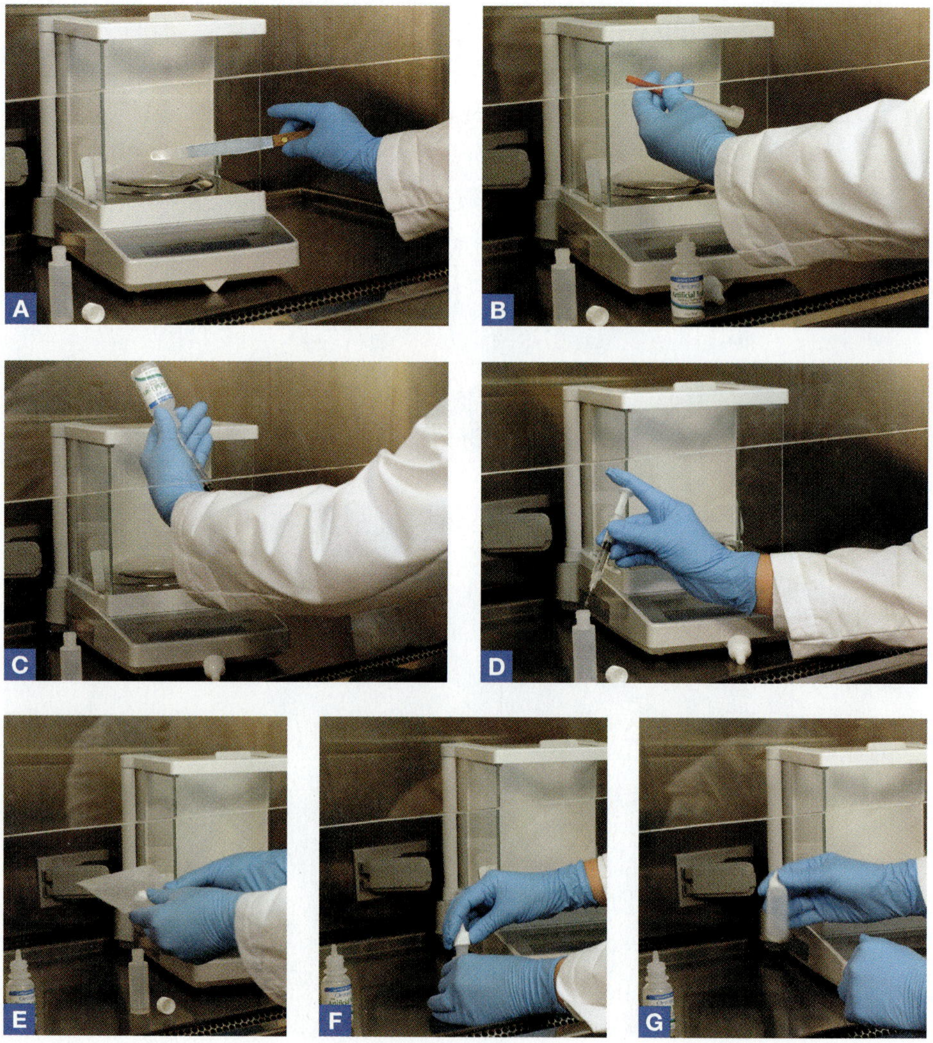

Figure 9-5 Compounding an ophthalmic solution/suspension

Suspensions

Dissolve the ingredients in about three-fourths of the total quantity of sterile water for injection, or a suitable diluent, and mix well. Add sufficient (QSAD) sterile water or diluent to the desired volume and mix well. Package in a suitable container for autoclaving. Autoclave, cool, and label. An autoclaved sample should be used for quality control testing. Alternatively, you can sterilize each ingredient by a suitable method. Then, under an LAFW or barrier isolator, using aseptic technique, dissolve the ingredients in about three-fourths of the quantity of sterile water for injection or suitable diluent and mix well. Add sufficient (QSAD) sterile water or diluent to the desired volume and mix well. Using a sterile needle and syringe, remove a sample of the suspension for quality control testing.

Ointments

Sterilize each ingredient by a suitable method, and then, under an LAFW or barrier isolator, using aseptic technique, mix the ingredients in the sterile vehicle. Take a sample of the ointment for quality control testing (Figure 9-6 A-N).

WORKPLACE WISDOM

If necessary, homogenize to reduce particle size and prepare a uniform suspension.

WORKPLACE WISDOM

Sift dry powders through a fine-screen sieve or mix in a dry powder pulverizer to reduce the particle size and eliminate clumps of powder.

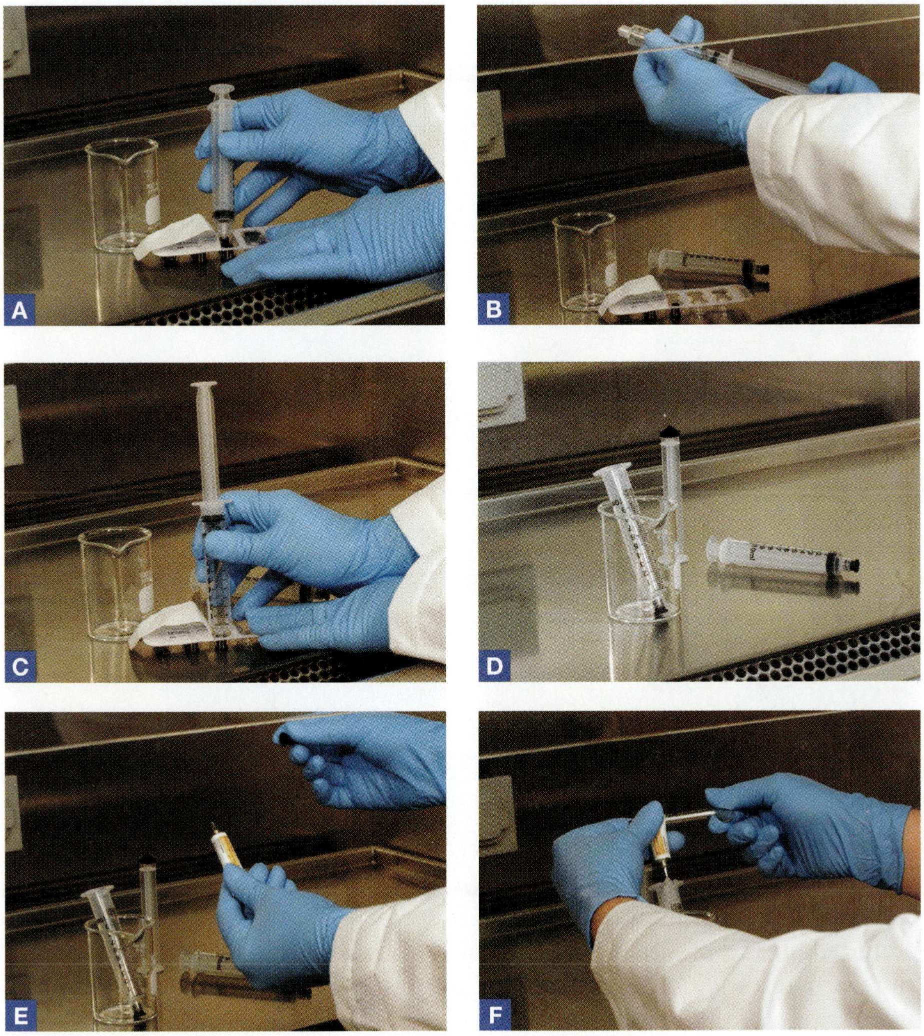

Figure 9-6 Compounding an ophthalmic ointment

Figure 9-6
Compounding an ophthalmic ointment (*continued*)

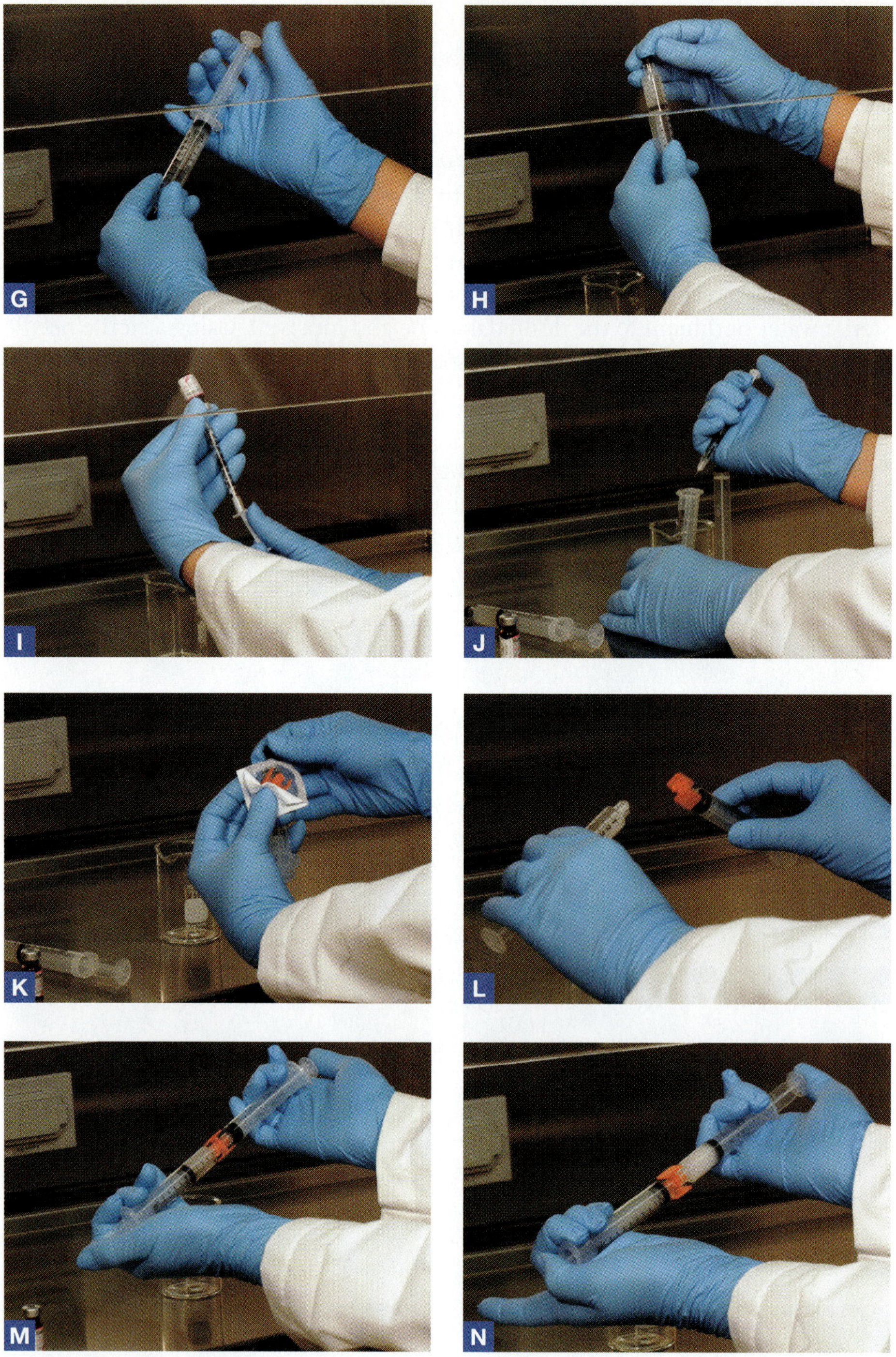

If all of the ingredients are sterile, all of the steps should be done under an LAFW or barrier isolator. If a large quantity or batch is being prepared, or if the beyond-use dating exceeds the USP 797 limits for untested compounded sterile products (CSPs), the product needs to be sterility tested and the batch should be quarantined until the sterility test comes back negative for growth.

QUALITY CONTROL

All weights, measurements, and final volumes should be double checked by the compounder and the pharmacist to ensure compounding accuracy and documented on the compounding worksheet. It is advisable to prepare extra product in order to take a sample for end-product testing. The sample should be taken after sterilization. A portion of the sample should be tested for sterility via the USP Direct Inoculation of the Culture Medium method or tested by a certified laboratory. The sample should be visually inspected using a lighted black and white background to check for clarity and particulate matter. The appearance should be as expected for the product with no unusual color or viscosity changes. The pH should be tested using a pH meter or pH paper to check if the product is within the acceptable pH range. Finally, the label should be checked for the proper information.

If the product was prepared in a batch and packaged in several containers to be dispensed to multiple patients, the batch should be quarantined or placed in a secure place until all end-product testing has been performed and passed. Since batch-compounded products have the potential to harm multiple patients, end-product testing is essential to ensure the integrity of the product and safety of the patients.

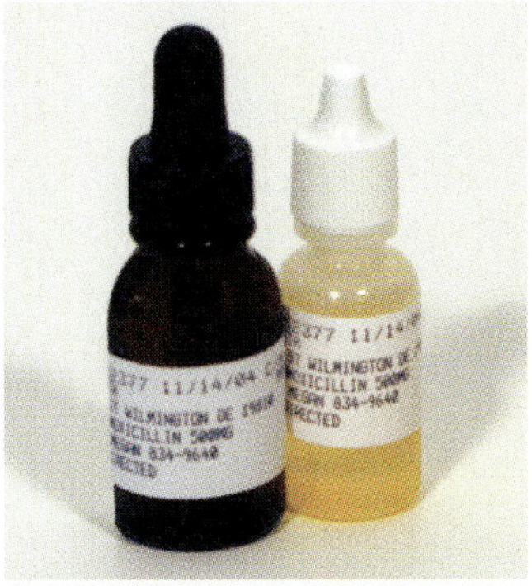

Figure 9-7 Packaged ophthalmic suspensions/solutions

PACKAGING

Ophthalmic solutions or suspensions should be packaged in sterile dropper bottles (Figure 9-7).They may be plastic or glass depending on the drug stability, but plastic is the most common. For drugs that are light sensitive, sterile amber dropper bottles should be used for dispensing, or the clear sterile dropper bottle should be placed in an amber vial and the patient instructed to store the preparation in the vial. Individual doses can also be placed in sterile, topical syringes or sterile syringes without needles. Ophthalmic ointments can also be placed in sterile syringes or sterile ophthalmic tubes.

LABELING

The following information should be included on all compounding labels: generic or chemical name of the active ingredient(s), strength and/or quantity, an assigned pharmacy lot number, beyond-use or expiration dating, storage requirements, and instructions for use.

All ophthalmic products should be labeled "For The Eye," "Do Not Touch the Eye or Eyelid," and "Discard after ____________." In appropriate instances, "Protect from Light" labels should be applied. Suspensions should also contain a "Shake Well" label (Figure 9-8).

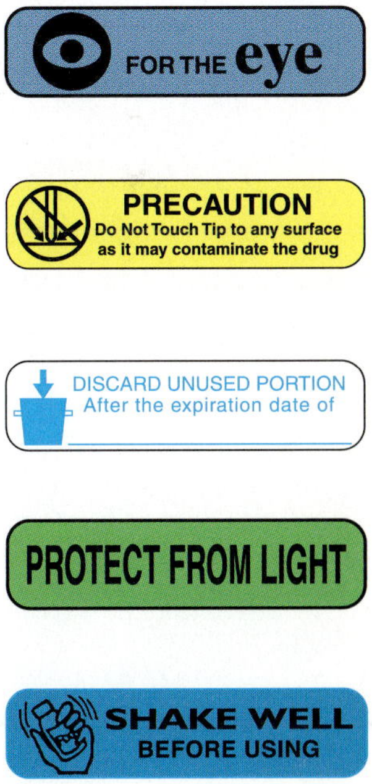

Figure 9-8 Auxiliary labels

STABILITY

Untested sterile ophthalmic preparations must be assigned expiration dates according to the appropriate risk levels described in the USP 797. Extended beyond-use dates may be used if supported by appropriate literature sources, such as published studies in journals, or by direct testing evidence. If no information is available, beyond-use dates are assigned as described in the section "Stability Criteria and Beyond-Use Dating" in the general test chapter "Pharmaceutical Compounding Nonsterile Preparations (795).

Aqueous or water-based solutions should be assigned a 14-day expiration date when stored at cold temperatures. Nonaqueous or oil-based liquids prepared with a manufactured product should be assigned an expiration date of six months or 25 percent of the manufacturer's expiration date, whichever is shorter. For all other products, a 30-day expiration date or the intended duration of therapy can be assigned, whichever is less.

PATIENT COUNSELING

The pharmacist should counsel patients on how to properly use the ophthalmic product. Ask the patient if he wants instruction or counseling from the pharmacist. When dispensing the ophthalmic preparation, instruct the patient about the storage requirements and caution him about not allowing the tip of the dropper or tube to touch anything, including the eye or eyelid.

Otic Dosage Forms

There are three types of otic dosage forms-solutions, suspensions, and powders.

TYPES AND DEFINITIONS

Solutions

Otic solutions are sterile liquid preparations that are clear because all of the ingredients are dissolved. They may be instilled in the ear or used as irrigations for the ear. Irrigation solutions can be warmed to about 37°C to improve patient comfort. They are useful in removing earwax, purulent discharges or pus from infections, and foreign objects from the ear.

Suspensions

Otic suspensions are sterile liquid preparations that contain visible insoluble ingredients. They are used to prolong a drug's effect if the drug is more viscous or if the drug cannot dissolve in a medium used for the ear.

Powders

Insufflations are fine powders, usually containing an antibacterial and/or antifungal, that are blown into the ear by using a rubber or plastic bulb called an insufflator or "puffer."

COMPOSITION AND INGREDIENTS

Common active ingredients used in otic preparations include local anesthetics, peroxides (cleansing agents), anti-infectives, and antifungals. Some liquids are used for cleaning, warming, or drying the external ear or ear canal and for removing debris.

The most common vehicles used in otic preparations are nonaqueous and are listed in Table 9-6

One of the therapeutic goals of otic preparations is to keep the ear canal dry to minimize bacterial and fungal growth. The nonaqueous vehicles are thick or viscous and will adhere to the ear canal. Water and alcohol (ethanol or isopropyl) can be used as vehicles, but are primarily used in otic irrigation solutions. Otic powders can contain talc or lactose as a vehicle or diluent, or they may be pure drug.

Unlike ophthalmics, hypertonicity is desired in otic preparations because excess or unwanted fluid moves from the inner ear canal into the outer ear canal where it will drain out, thus releasing pressure and discomfort that the patient can experience with ear infections.

Inefficient cleaning of the ear commonly causes ear problems. **Surfactants** are added to otic preparations to evenly distribute the drug when administered and to help break up earwax. This action makes it easier to clean and irrigate the ear by removing the foreign debris.

Many of the nonaqueous vehicles are concentrated and self-preserving, such as glycerin and propylene glycol. Since these vehicles are commonly used, many otic preparations do not require preservatives. Aqueous solutions may require a preservative (Table 9-1) if they are intended for multiple use.

TABLE 9-6 Nonaqueous Vehicles Used in Otic Preparations

Glycerin
Propylene Glycol
Lower Weight Polyethylene Glycols (PEGs)
Vegetable Oils
Mineral Oil

surfactants
a surface-active substance

PREPARATION AND COMPOUNDING TECHNIQUES

Until January 2004, otic products needed to be prepared in a "clean" environment, such as ISO Class 8 or Class 100,000. According to the USP 797, otic preparations are now considered sterile products and must be prepared accordingly.

Solutions

Dissolve the ingredients in about three-fourths of the total quantity of the vehicle and mix well. Add sufficient (QSAD) vehicle to the desired volume and mix well. Under an LAFW or barrier isolator, using aseptic technique, filter the solution through a sterile 0.2 micron membrane filter into a sterile container. Using a sterile needle and syringe, remove a sample of the solution for quality control testing (Figure 9-9 A-I).

Suspensions

After having all measured ingredients double checked, dissolve the ingredients in about three-fourths the total quantity of the vehicle and mix well. Add sufficient (QSAD) vehicle to the desired volume and mix well. Package in a suitable container for sterilization, then sterilize using a suitable method, cool, and label. Extract a sterile sample for quality control testing. Alternatively, sterilize each ingredient by a suitable method, and then, under an LAFW or barrier isolator, using aseptic technique, dissolve the ingredients in about three-fourths of the quantity of sterile water for injection or suitable diluent and mix well. Add sufficient (QSAD) sterile water or diluent to the desired volume and mix well. Using a sterile needle and syringe, remove a sample of the suspension for quality control testing.

Figure 9-9
Compounding an otic solution/suspension

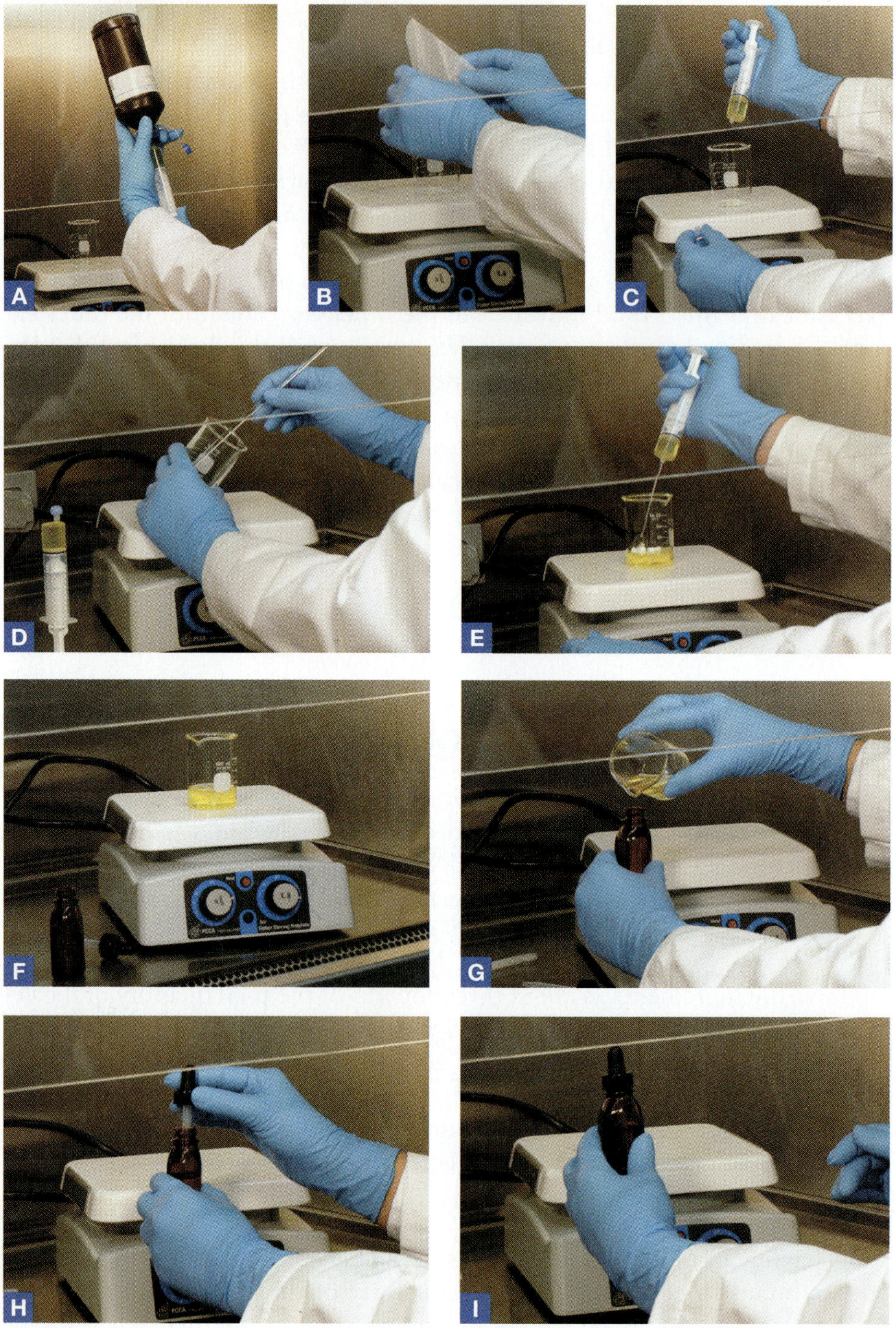

Ointments

Sterilize each ingredient by a suitable method. Then, under an LAFW, using aseptic technique, mix each ingredient into the vehicle. Take a sample of the ointment for quality control testing (Figure 9-10 A-N).

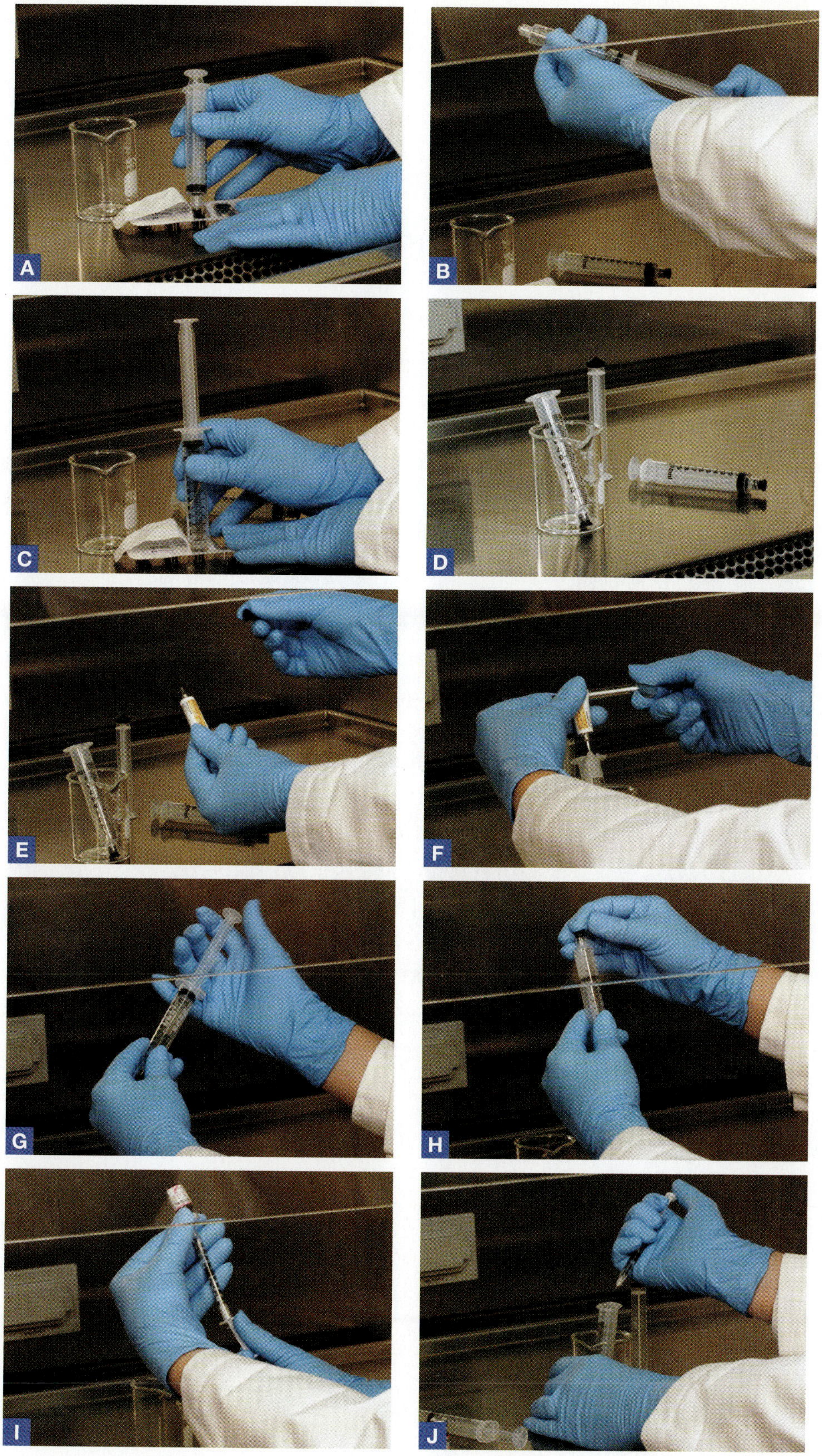

Figure 9-10
Compounding an otic ointment

Figure 9-10
Compounding an otic ointment (*continued*)

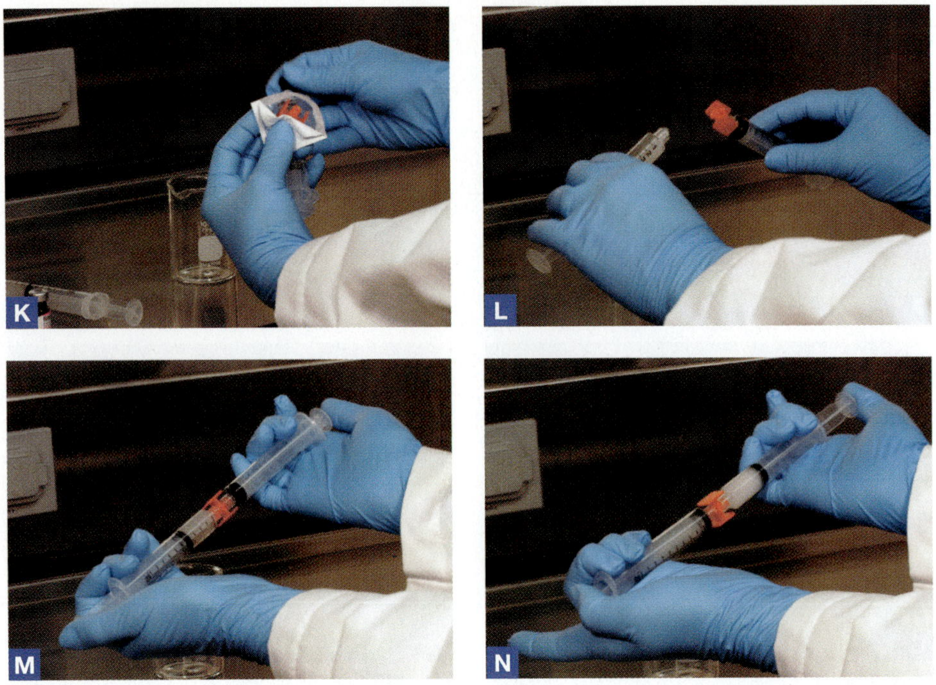

Powders

Sterilize each ingredient by a suitable method. Then, under an LAFW, using aseptic technique, geometrically mix powders together, starting with the powders present in the smallest quantity. Take a sample of the powder for quality control testing (Figure 9-11 A-J).

Figure 9-11
Compounding an otic powder

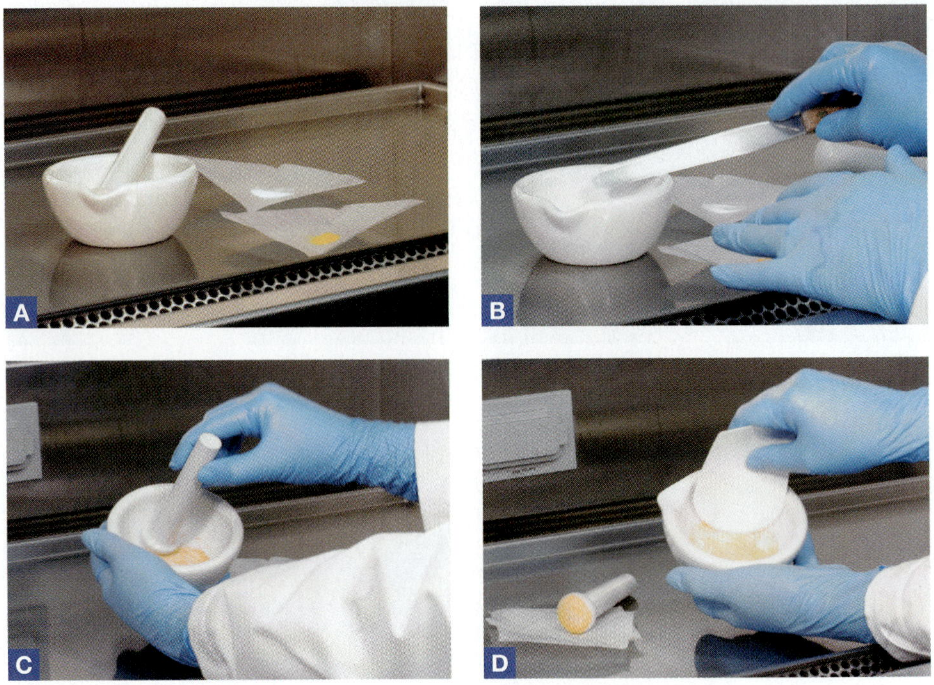

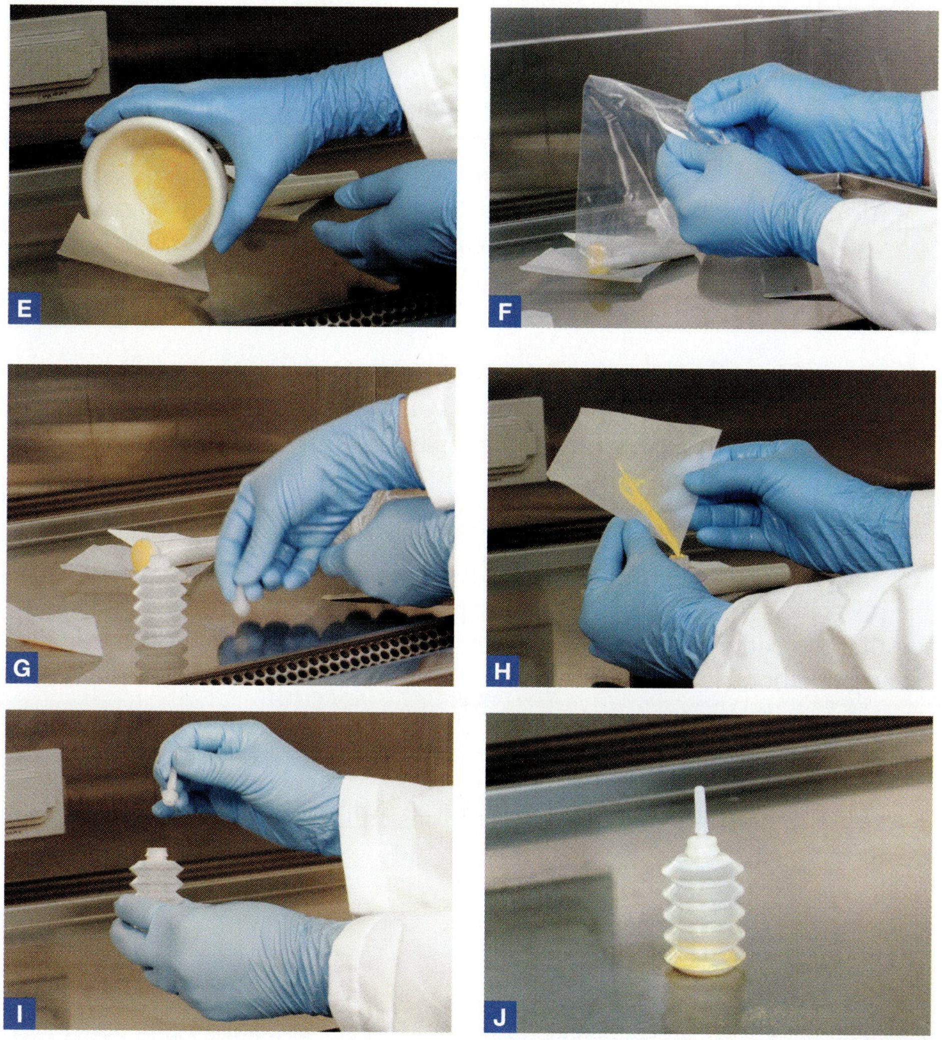

Figure 9-11 Compounding an otic powder (*continued*)

Again, if all of the ingredients are sterile, all of the steps should be done under an LAFW or barrier isolator. If a large quantity or batch is being prepared or the beyond-use dating exceeds the USP 797 limits for untested compounded sterile products (CSPs), the product needs to be sterility tested and the batch should be quarantined until the sterility test comes back negative for growth.

QUALITY CONTROL

All otic preparations should be double checked, sterility tested, and pH tested in the same manner as the ophthalmic preparations. Batch-compounded otic products are also done in the same manner as the ophthalmic preparations. Additionally, otic preparations should be visually and physically checked for viscosity and appearance.

PACKAGING

Otic solutions or suspensions, like ophthalmic preparations, should be packaged in dropper containers. Otic ointments should be packaged in sterile tubes or sterile syringes and otic powders in insufflators or "puffers" (Figure 9-12).

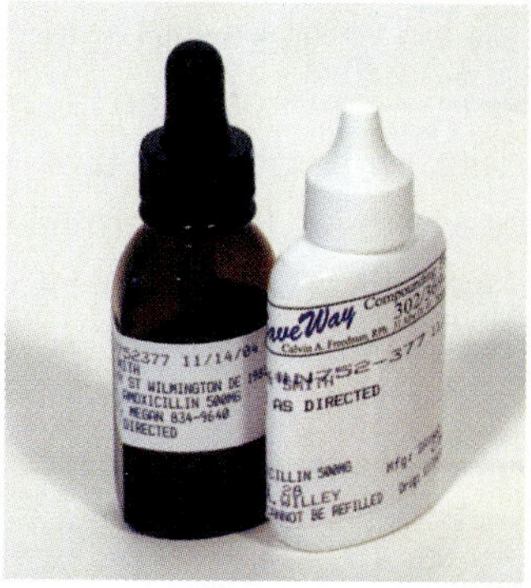

Figure 9-12 Packaged otic preparations

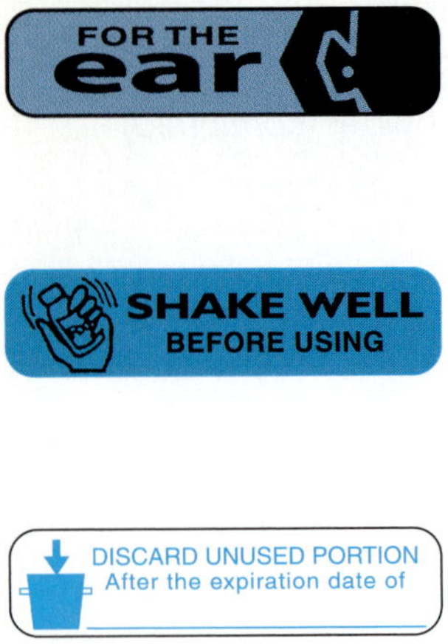

Figure 9-13 Auxiliary labels

LABELING

The following information should be included on all compounding labels: generic or chemical name of the active ingredient(s), strength and/or quantity, an assigned pharmacy lot number, beyond-use or expiration dating, storage requirements, and instructions for use.

All otic preparations should be labeled "For the Ear" and "Discard after __________." Suspensions should contain a "Shake Well" label, too (Figure 9-13).

STABILITY

All otic products can be stored at either room temperature or refrigerated, but never frozen. The expiration or beyond-use date is determined in the same manner as that for ophthalmic preparations.

PATIENT COUNSELING

Ask the patient if he would like to receive counseling and/or instruction from the pharmacist on how to use the otic preparation. Make sure when dispensing that the patient knows how to store the product. The patient should also be reminded not to touch the tip of the dropper or tube on the ear.

Nasal Dosage Forms

There are three types of nasal dosage forms-solutions and supensions, ointments, and gels.

TYPES AND DEFINITIONS

Solutions and Suspensions

Nasal solutions are sterile, clear liquids and nasal suspensions are sterile liquids that contain visible insoluble ingredients. Both types of dosage forms are administered as drops or sprays in the nose. These products may be intended for either local or systemic use.

WORKPLACE WISDOM

Mineral oil should never be used in nasal preparations. It has been proven to be harmful if introduced or inhaled into the respiratory system.

Ointments

Nasal ointments and gels are sterile, semi-solid preparations that are applied in the nose via a swab. They may have a local or systemic drug effect.

Gels

Nasal gels are aqueous-based, whereas nasal ointments are usually nonaqueous-based.

COMPOSITION AND INGREDIENTS

Nasal preparations are very similar in composition to ophthalmic preparations. In addition to the active ingredients, nasal products require several different ingredients: vehicles, buffers, preservatives, tonicity agents, gelling agents, and antioxidants.

The vehicle should have a pH range of 4–8 with a mild buffer capacity. The nasal fluid is also isotonic, similar to 0.9 percent sodium chloride solution. Tonicity values can range from 0.6 to 1.8 percent sodium chloride equivalency or 200 to 600 mOsm/L , with 300 mOsm/L being the optimum value. If the tonicity falls out of range, the nasal ciliary movement can slow or stop. Otic preparations must be in the proper pH and tonicity ranges to be nonirritating and compatible with the nose.

PREPARATION AND COMPOUNDING TECHNIQUES

Solutions

As with all compounds, accurately weigh or measure each ingredient and have the quantities double checked. Dissolve the ingredients in about three-fourths of the total quantity of sterile water for injection or suitable diluent and mix well. Add sufficient (QSAD) sterile water or diluent to the desired volume and mix well. Under an LAFW or barrier isolator, using aseptic technique, filter the solution through a sterile 0.2 micron filter into a sterile ophthalmic container. Using a sterile needle and syringe, remove a sample of the solution for quality control testing (Figure 9-14 A-K).

Suspensions

Dissolve the ingredients in about three-fourths of the total quantity of sterile water for injection or suitable diluent and mix well. Add sufficient (QSAD) sterile water or diluent to the desired volume and mix well. Package in a suitable container for autoclaving, then autoclave, cool, and label. Use an autoclaved sample for quality

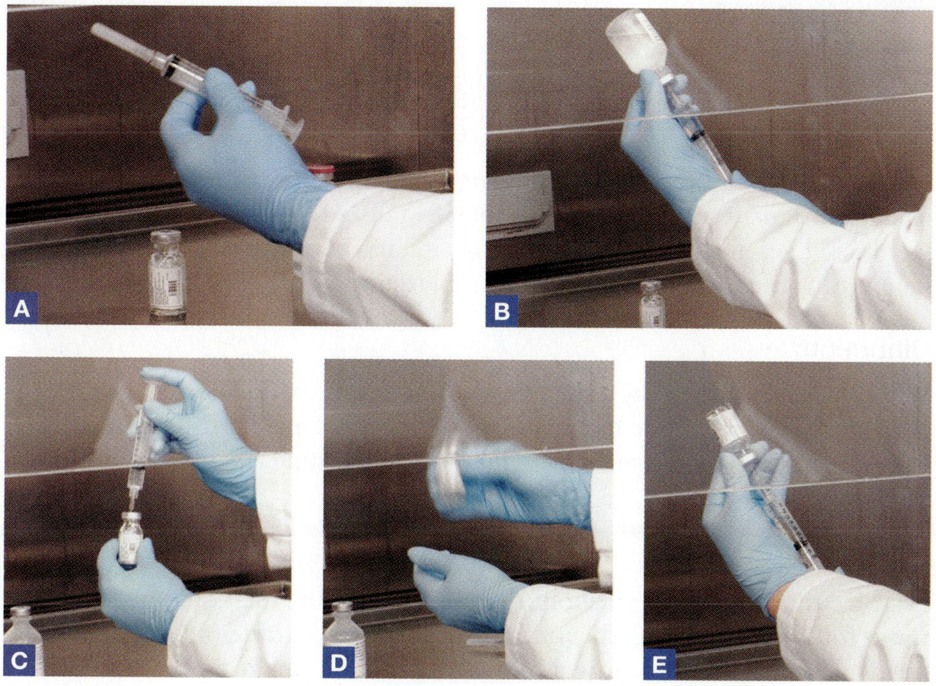

Figure 9-14
Compounding a nasal solution/suspension

Figure 9-14
Compounding a nasal solution/suspension (*continued*)

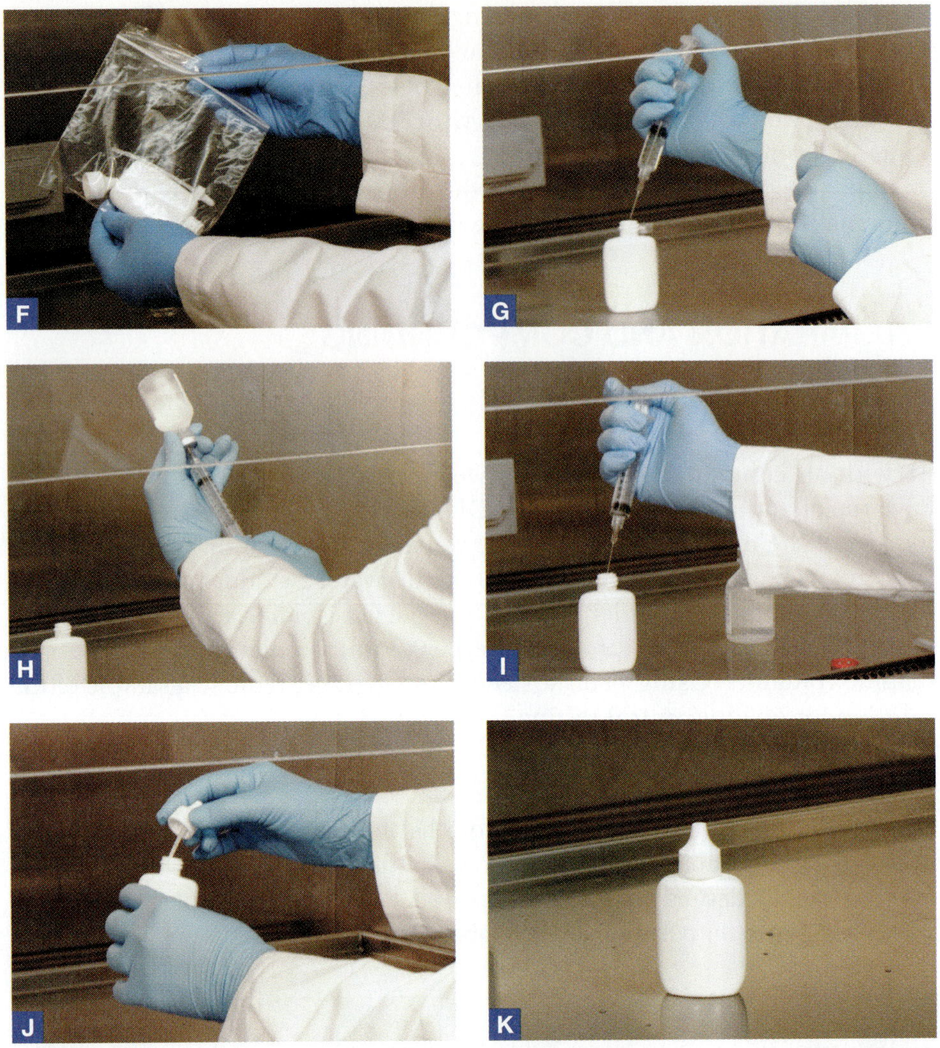

control testing. Alternatively, sterilize each ingredient by a suitable method, and then, under an LAFW or barrier isolator, using aseptic technique, dissolve the ingredients in about three-fourths of the total quantity of sterile water for injection or suitable diluent and mix well. Add sufficient (QSAD) sterile water or diluent to the desired volume and mix well. Using a sterile needle and syringe, remove a sample of the suspension for quality control testing.

Ointments

Sterilize each ingredient by a suitable method, and then, under an LAFW or barrier isolator, using aseptic technique, mix the ingredients in the sterile vehicle. Take a sample of the ointment for quality control testing (Figure 9-15 A-H).

GELS

Dissolve the ingredients in about three-fourths of the total quantity of sterile water for injection or suitable diluent and mix well. Under an LAFW or barrier isolator, using aseptic technique, filter solution through a 0.2 micron

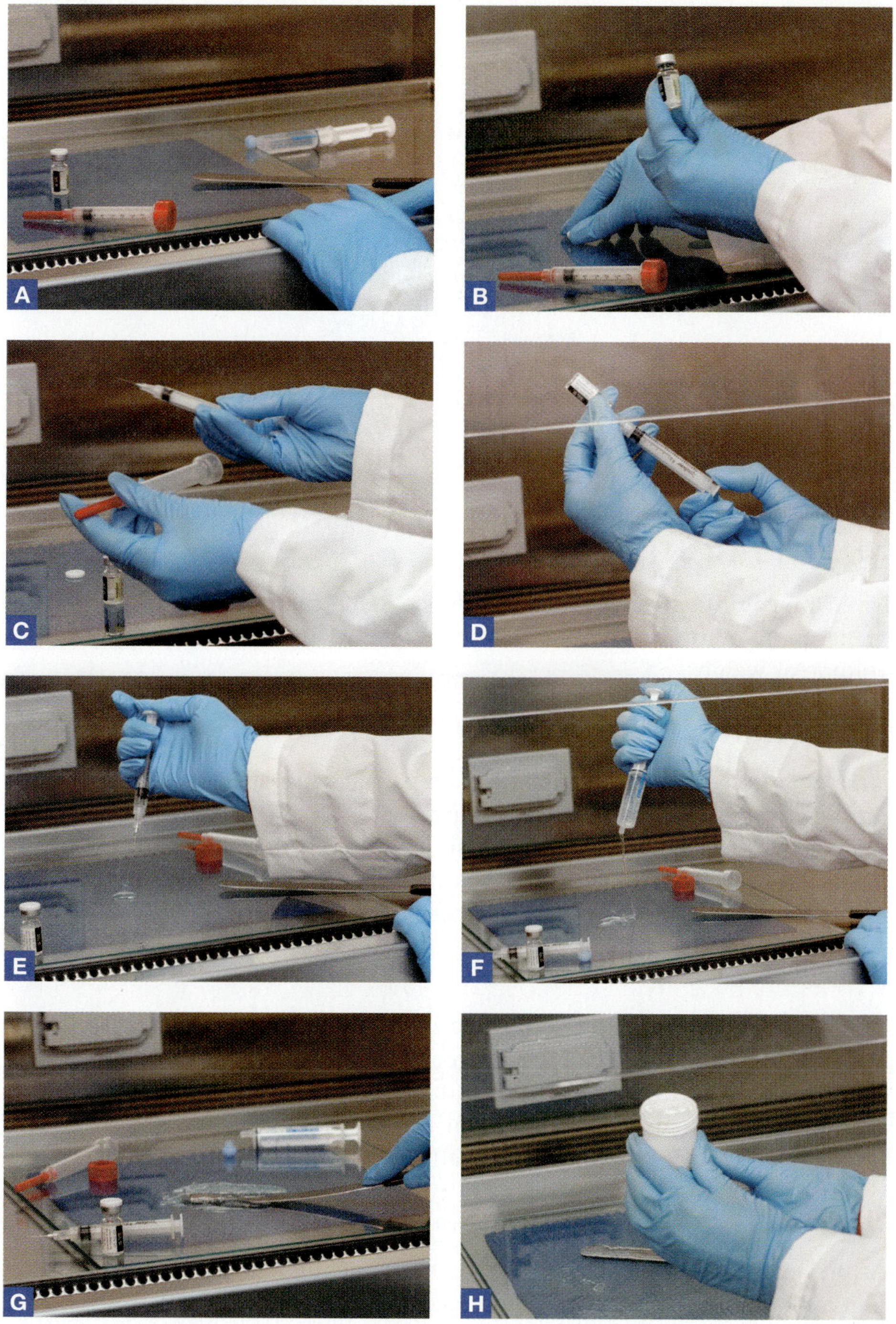

Figure 9-15
Compounding a nasal ointment/gel

membrane filter into a sterile container. Add the gelling agent (previously sterilized) and mix well. Add sufficient (QSAD) sterile water for injection to the desired volume or weight and mix well.

As stated before, if all of the ingredients are sterile, all of the steps should be done under an LAFW or barrier isolator. If a large quantity or batch is being prepared or the beyond-use dating exceeds the USP 797 limits for untested compounded sterile products (CSPs), the product needs to be

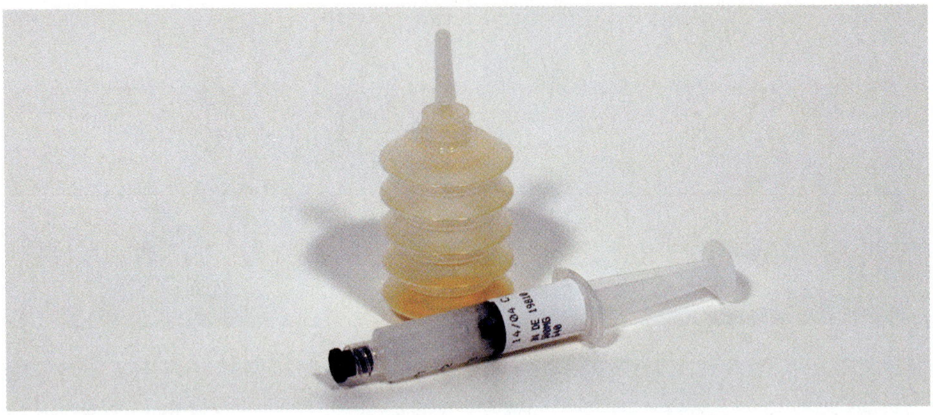

Figure 9-16 Packaged nasal preparations

sterility tested and the batch should be quarantined until the sterility test comes back negative for growth.

QUALITY CONTROL

Nasal preparations must be tested in the same manner as the ophthalmic preparations. Procedures should include testing for sterility, clarity, pH, and volume or weight.

PACKAGING

Nasal solutions and suspensions can be packaged in sterile, plastic or glass, dropper bottles or spray bottles (Figure 9-16). Metered spray bottles deliver a consistent, specific dose per spray and are used primarily when the drug is to be absorbed systemically. Nasal ointments and gels may be individually packaged as single doses in sterile tubes.

LABELING

The following information should be included on all compounding labels: generic or chemical name of the active ingredient(s), strength and/or quantity, an assigned pharmacy lot number, beyond-use or expiration dating, storage requirements, and instructions for use. All nasal preparations should be labeled "For the Nose" and "Discard after ____________" (Figure 9-17).

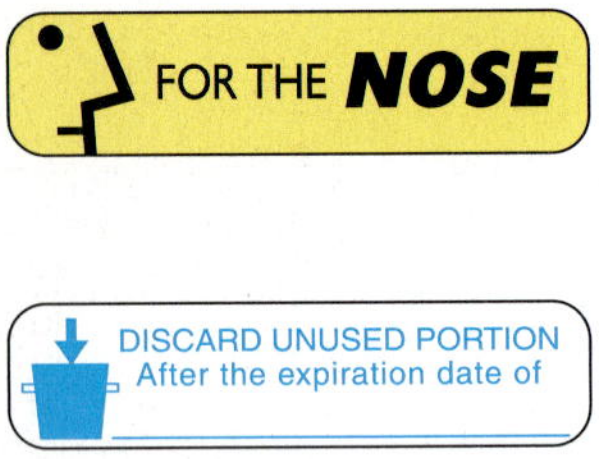

Figure 9-17 Auxiliary labels

STABILITY

As previously discussed in the Section on ophthalmic preparations, the expiration or beyond-use date is determined according to the USP standards. All nasal preparations may be stored at room temperature or refrigerated, but not frozen.

PATIENT COUNSELING

Ask the patient if he would like counseling by the pharmacist about the medication or on how to use the nasal preparation. If the drug is intended to be systemically absorbed or absorbed into the bloodstream, the patient should be counseled on possible side effects of the drug(s). Before dispensing the preparation, inform the patient about the storage requirements.

SUMMARY

Most extemporaneously compounded prescriptions are prepared in a non-sterile, but clean, environment and do not require the practice of aseptic technique. Ophthalmic, otic, and nasal preparations, however, do require both a sterile environment and the use of proper aseptic technique. While this chapter has reviewed these dosage forms in the same format as the chapters on capsules, liquids, gels, and the like, it has not described aseptic technique. To be qualified to prepare the compounds described in this chapter, you must study and practice aseptic technique first.

PROFILES OF PRACTICE

Sample Formula: Artificial Tears

for training purposes only

Polyvinyl alcohol	1.5 ml
Povidone	0.5 ml
Chlorobutanol	0.5 ml
Normal Saline (sterile)	97.5 ml

1. Accurately measure each ingredient.
2. Dissolve all ingredients in the normal saline.
3. Filter through a 0.2 micron filter into a sterile ophthalmic container.
4. Package and label.

Sample Formula: Saline Mist (Nasal)

for training purposes only

Sodium chloride	650 mg
Monobasic potassium phosphate	40 mg
Dibasic potassium phosphate	90 mg
Benzalkonium chloride	10 mg
Sterile water	qs

1. Accurately measure each ingredient.
2. Dissolve the ingredients in enough sterile water to make 100 ml of solution.
3. Filter through a 0.2 micron filter into a sterile container.
4. Package and label.

CHAPTER TERMS

autoclaved
a method of sterilization where heat is used

filtration
the passage of a liquid through a filter to sterilize or remove foreign particles

surfactants
a surface-active substance

tonicity
a state of normal tension of the tissues by virtue of which the parts are kept in shape, alert, and ready to function in response to a suitable stimulus

viscosity
a physical property of fluids that determines the internal resistance to shear forces

CHAPTER 9

CHAPTER REVIEW QUESTIONS

1. Why are surfactants added to otic preparations?
   a. to help the mixture flow easy
   b. to help break up the earwax
   c. as a buffer for sufficient quantity
   d. for a preservative-free mixture

2. Otic preparations can never be stored
   a. at room temperature
   b. in the refrigerator
   c. in the freezer
   d. both a and b

3. A product used in ophthalmic preparations to maintain the pH of the product within the desired range during the storage and administration in the eye is known as
   a. a buffer
   b. a surfactant
   c. mineral oil
   d. PEG

4. When should a sample be taken from a compounded batch?
   a. when the first liquid ingredient is incorporated
   b. after sterilization
   c. after levigation takes place
   d. before the dry ingredients are added

5. A nasal preparation should be in the pH range of
   a. 4–8
   b. 7–10
   c. 4–6
   d. 3–5

6. True or false: Mineral oil should never be used in nasal preparations because it has been proven to be harmful to the respiratory system.
   a. true
   b. false

7. True or false: Viscosity refers to the physical properties of fluids that determine the internal resistance to shear forces.
   a. true
   b. false

8. Why is hypertonicity desired in otic preparations?

9. List the requirements for information that must be on a compounded label.

10. **Critical Thinking** Why do ophthalmic, otic, and nasal preparations require sterile environments and aseptic technique?

Resources and References

1. Allen, Loyd V, Jr., Ph.D. *The Art, Science, and Technology of Pharmaceutical Compounding*. Washington, DC: American Pharmaceutical Association, 1998.
2. Pharmaceutical Compounding–Sterile Preparations In: *United States Pharmacopeia 27/National Formulary* 22. Rockville, MD: United States Pharmacopeial Convention, 2003.
3. Sterility Tests (71) In: *United States Pharmacopeia 27/National Formulary* 22. Rockville, MD: United States Pharmacopeial Convention, 2003.
4. Stability Criteria and Beyond-Use Dating—Pharmaceutical Compounding Nonsterile Preparations (795) In: *United States Pharmacopeia 27/National Formulary* 22. Rockville, MD: United States Pharmacopeial Convention, 2003.

CHAPTER 10

Medication Flavoring

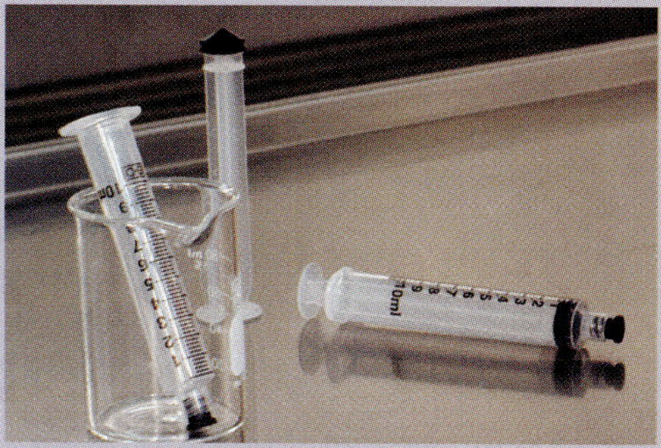

Learning Objectives

After completing this chapter, you should be able to:

- Describe the proper excipients and techniques used in flavoring medications.
- List the various properties of chemicals, flavoring agents, sweetening agents, suspending agents, diluting agents, and coloring agents.
- Define different patient types and individual drug classes and recommend the most appropriate flavor choices for each group.

INTRODUCTION

Successfully flavoring a medication is a critical step in the process of properly preparing a prescription, especially when the taste of a particular drug is such that it will not be tolerated by the patient when administered orally.

Psychological Impact

Although no **therapeutic** benefit is evident, using the proper coloring and flavoring for medicinal substances is of considerable importance psychologically. A liquid medication that is as clear as water and has no smell to it will be thought by the patient or the caregiver to lack the active ingredient(s). Conversely, a liquid that has been flavored, for example, with bubblegum and slightly tinged with a pink color will be thought to be more effective. A medication that is disagreeable in either appearance, texture, or taste can be made more attractive and **palatable** by the careful choice of the most appropriate flavoring, sweetening, diluting, suspending, or coloring agent. The selection of the proper agent is important in preparing the best formulation and in ensuring patient compliance when administering the medication.

therapeutic
a desired effect pertaining to the art of healing

palatable
pleasing to the taste

SENSORY ROLES IN FLAVORING

Taste, smell, sight, touch, and even sound are complex experiences that may influence the flavor sensation. In general, individuals are usually more sensitive to the aroma of a preparation than to the actual taste. Elderly patients may require added amounts of flavor in order to achieve the desired result. Females tend to be more sensitive to smell than males are. Certain diseases will alter a patient's ability to taste and smell. For example, a patient suffering from a cold or influenza may have a dulled sense of smell and/or taste. When the nostrils are held closed, raw onions will taste sweet, and likewise, nauseating smelling medications will be much easier to ingest.

Psychological factors such as sight and sound play an important role in flavor experience when certain reflexes become conditioned through association. As in the classic experiments of Pavlov, the ringing of the bell caused the gastric juices of a dog to flow, even though there was no food placed in front of it. Part of the enjoyment of eating crunchy foods such as raw celery or carrots is the sound they make as they are being chewed. Furthermore, the color of a preparation and the flavor should coincide. For example, cherry flavored substances should be red and grape substances should be purple.

Flavoring Considerations

idiosyncrasies
unusual individual reactions to food or a drug

Each prescription that presents itself for flavoring must be considered on an individual basis. It is important to be aware of any allergies or sensitivities a patient may have to particular ingredients, such as chocolate, peanuts, or possibly a particular preservative or dye. It is also helpful to know the likes and dislikes as well as any **idiosyncrasies** a patient may have. One should not rely on what is traditionally used or a flavor choice that is popular among a select group. Although most pediatric patients like flavors such as grape, bubblegum, or cherry, some patients may not tolerate the tannins or a specific dye contained in the flavoring agent, or they simply may not care for these flavors.

PEDIATRIC FLAVORING

Children have more taste buds than adults and therefore are more sensitive to taste. Infants and children tend to prefer tastes that are sweet and do not respond well to bitter flavors. Appropriate flavor choices for children include raspberry, bubblegum, marshmallow, butterscotch, citrus, berry, and vanilla. The palate of a newborn or an infant typically has not been exposed to a wide variety of tastes; therefore, this young patient will not require as strong a flavor as an older patient. A patient who is required to take a medication for a long period of time may require a milder flavor in order to avoid flavor fatigue.

ADULT FLAVORING

Adults are usually more tolerant of a bitter flavor, so with extremely bitter drugs, a flavoring agent such as coffee, chocolate, cherry, anise, grapefruit, or mint will be acceptable. These bitter flavors are generally an acquired taste. Their own "bite" is helpful in cutting the bitterness of the drug.

IMPACT ON STABILITY, SOLUBILITY, AND pH

Other factors to be considered when choosing an appropriate flavoring agent include stability, solubility, pH, and the physical properties of the flavors available. Some flavors will cause a negative effect in the compounded prescription, such as raising or lowering the pH of the final product, possibly causing instability. *Aqueous solutions* should be flavored with water **miscible** flavors, whereas oil preparations will require the flavor to be oil-based. These factors may limit a patient's choice of available flavors. Some flavoring agents or the preservatives contained within may affect the active ingredient, causing degradation of the drug.

miscible
susceptible to being mixed

Compounded medications that are stable only at a certain pH should be flavored with an agent that will not affect the pH or one that will enhance the pH of the final product. Although pH values may be equal to or within close range from manufacturer to manufacturer, the exact pH should be obtained from the company that is the source of the flavoring agent. Most chemical companies that offer products for medicinal flavoring will be able to provide a list of their flavors and the relative pH values. This is a reference that every pharmacy that offers flavoring as a service should have.

Four Taste Types

There are four basic taste experiences: sour, sweet, bitter, and salty. Each of these four taste types is experienced in a specific area of the tongue that contains taste buds with specialized functions. Taste **receptors** for all tastes are located in a narrow area surrounding the entire tongue. Sweet, salty, and sour taste receptors are in a region just inside the outer edge of the tongue. Salty and sour receptors are located in a small region toward the back of the tongue. Sour-only receptors are located approximately in the center of the tongue. There is an area toward the center and front of the tongue where no sensation of taste is experienced. Sweet and sour taste receptors are located just in front of this region with bittersweet and sour tastes being experienced near the tip of the tongue just inside the area containing the receptors for all tastes (Figure 10-1). The brain, however, is not able to discern between different taste components, but rather perceives taste as a composite sensation.

receptors
a molecular structure within a cell or on the surface characterized by selective binding of a specific substance and a specific physiologic effect that accompanies the binding

Physical Properties

When attempting to derive a good-tasting product, the properties of the chemicals and any excipients in the formula should be taken into consideration. A hot taste due to a mild counterirritant effect may be covered by using a flavor with similar properties, such as cinnamon, wintergreen, or teaberry. Sour taste is caused by hydrogen ions and is characteristic of acids, tannins,

Figure 10-1 Four basic taste experiences

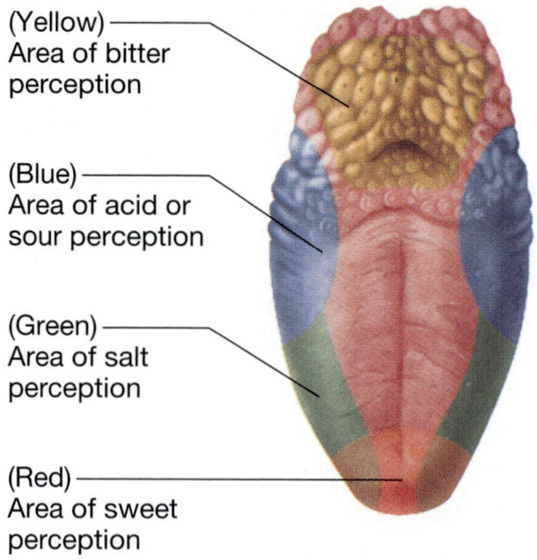

and lactones. Raspberry syrup is effective in masking sour tastes, whereas acacia syrup will disguise the sour taste by forming a protective coating over the taste buds of the tongue. A cooling sensation is due to a negative heat of a solution. This property can be overcome by using flavors that likewise give off a cooling effect such as wintergreen, mint, or teaberry. Preservatives also have characteristics that may affect flavoring.

Grittiness of the final preparation should be avoided. This may be achieved by properly reducing particle size, thoroughly dissolving the ingredients in the proper vehicle, or by homogenizing the final product. Grittiness may also be due to the texture of the drug or an excipient and may or may not be prevented depending on the nature of these ingredients. If grittiness does exist in the final product, the patient should be instructed not to "chew" the particles, but to swallow them whole.

Flavoring Techniques

Flavoring medications can be seen as both a challenge and an opportunity. The challenge is in the fact that there are no general or definite rules for what is right. There are no absolutes when it comes to flavoring, especially when working with an extemporaneously compounded prescription. Every formula that requires flavoring should be analyzed individually. The challenge of flavoring is further complicated by the individual preferences of each patient. The opportunity in flavoring lies in the ability to produce a quality product that the patient is willing to take or, at the very least, the patient will tolerate.

There are five basic flavoring techniques used when preparing an acceptable product that minimizes a negative experience with regard to taste.

1. **Blending** uses a flavor that will blend with the drug taste. Citrus flavors blend with sour tastes; bitter tastes can be blended with salty, sweet, and sour tastes; salt reduces bitterness and sourness and increases sweetness. Chemicals such as vanillin, monosodium glutamate, and benzaldehyde are used for blending.

2. **Overshadowing** or overpowering involves the use of a flavor with a stronger intensity than the original product. Examples of intense flavoring vehicles are wintergreen, methyl salicylate, glycyrrhiza (licorice), and oleoresins.

3. **Physical methods** include the formulation of insoluble ingredients into a suspension; emulsification of oils—where the offensive-tasting ingredient is placed in the oil phase and the flavoring or sweetening agent is placed in the aqueous phase. Effervescent additives are used in the preparation of salty-tasting drugs. The use of a high-viscosity fluid such as a syrup will limit contact of the offensive element with the tongue.

4. **Chemical methods** include absorbing the drug with an ingredient that eliminates the taste of the offensive drug.

5. **Physiological methods** involve using an additive such as menthol, peppermint, spearmint or a spice such as cinnamon or clove to anesthetize the taste buds within the tongue. These flavor products will reduce the sensitivity of the taste buds to bitterness.

In addition, *flavor enhancers*, such as a monosodium glutamate, may be added to ensure intensity of flavor. The most used flavor enhancer is vanilla. It can be added along with almost any flavoring agent to stimulate and intensify the desired flavor without altering the flavor or adding its own taste.

WORKPLACE WISDOM

Another flavor enhancing choice to consider is marshmallow. Marshmallow will intensify sweet tastes as well as give the deception of a sweeter taste. It is especially effective when compounding bitter drugs.

Tastes Needing Flavoring

There are four main categories of taste that present as a flavor which may need to be masked. The syrups that are recommended for compounding these flavor sensations, as well as suggested flavoring choices for each, are listed as follows:

1. **Salty taste**—A salty taste is best hidden in cinnamon syrup. Other syrups used are, in descending order of effectiveness, orange syrup, citric acid syrup, cherry syrup, cocoa syrup, raspberry syrup, and glycyrrhiza syrup. Glycyrrhiza syrup is particularly useful because of its natural sweetness coupled with the sweetness of the sucrose in the syrup, and because of its ability to coat both the drug and the tongue, preventing contact. Suggested flavoring choices are nut, butterscotch, spice, and maple.

2. **Bitter taste**—Cocoa syrup is usually the best choice for covering bitter drugs, followed by raspberry syrup, cherry syrup, cinnamon syrup, citrus syrup, anise syrup, orange syrup, and wild cherry syrup. Suggested

flavoring choices are licorice, coffee, chocolate, mint, grapefruit, cherry, peach, raspberry, orange, lemon, and lime.

3. **Sour taste**—Raspberry syrup and other fruit syrups are especially effective in covering the taste of sour substances. Acacia syrup is also effective, depending on the drug, because it tends to coat the drug as well as the tongue, preventing the taste buds from coming in contact with the offending substance. Tragacanth is useful when working with alcoholic-based vehicles. Suggested flavoring choices are lemon, lime, orange, cherry, grapefruit, raspberry, and acacia.

4. **Oily taste**—Cod liver oil can be effectively disguised by using peppermint or wintergreen oil. Lemon, orange, and anise are other choices appropriate for this product. When compounding an oil product, it is best to choose a fixed oil base that contains no distinct flavor, such as sweet almond oil, which is easily flavored by adding any oil-based flavor choice. Suggested flavoring choices are peppermint, anise, wintergreen, teaberry, and cinnamon.

Simply adding a flavoring or coloring agent to a dosage form will not guarantee that a bad-tasting drug will taste good. An equally important element in flavoring a prescription is the sweetening agent. A *sweetening agent* must be used in order for the preparation to be palatable and acceptable to the patient. *Flavoring agents* are not sweet; in fact, they are quite bitter and therefore do not mask offensive-tasting drugs when used alone. The added flavor will simply give the aroma and taste of the added flavor. If a flavoring agent alone is added, it may actually make the preparation more bitter. Also, if too much of a flavoring is added, it can make an otherwise palatable formulation become bitter.

Sweeteners

There are a number of products used to sweeten compounded prescriptions. Some of the most commonly used are sucrose, dextrose, corn syrup, sorbitol, mannitol, and combinations of other sugars. Sweetening products such as Ora-Sweet®, Karo® Syrup, and simple syrup are widely used in the preparation of oral liquids. Since the viscosity of highly concentrated sugar solutions may slow down the rate of dissolution of a drug, it is advisable to dissolve the active ingredient and excipients in an aqueous vehicle before combining them with the sweetening agent. There are several noncalorie sweeteners, such as saccharin, aspartame, asulfame, and stevia that may be used when compounding prescriptions. It is important to know their physical properties, such as aftertaste, temperature sensitivity, pH sensitivity, and sweetening ability. Each sweetener has a unique sweetening ability, and the amount required should be calculated accordingly.

General Practices

The general rule for flavoring liquids is that water miscible flavors are added to aqueous formulations, and oil flavors are used when the liquid serving as the base is a fixed oil. There may be an instance where an oil flavoring must be added to an aqueous product. This can be done by dissolving the oil flavoring agent in a small amount of glycerin or sorbitol and then incorporating it into the liquid. This technique can also accomplish the task of adding an oily drug to such dosage forms as lollipops, lozenges, or gummy type bases.

Diluting Agents

Diluting agents are inactive substances used as solvents for drugs, but primarily for diluting and/or flavoring liquid medications intended for oral use. There are four basic kinds of diluting agents, differentiated by their physical properties: fixed oils, aqueous, hydroalcoholic, and alcoholic.

FIXED-OIL DILUTING AGENTS

A fixed oil is used as a diluting vehicle when a drug is oil soluble. A fixed oil may also be used if a drug may be unstable due to hydrolysis. A perfect example of this type of drug is aspirin. Oils are also an excellent choice with regard to flavoring because of their coating ability, which prevents contact of the drug with the taste buds. Cod liver oil is a fixed oil and serves as an excellent choice for dogs, cats, and other fish- or liver-loving animals. Since it has a very strong flavor, it may be advisable to dilute it by as much as 50 percent with another fixed oil that has little or no flavor or smell.

There are several commercially available fixed-oil products used regularly in the compounding pharmacy. These include sweet oil, peanut oil, corn oil, mineral oil, sesame oil, and sweet almond oil. There is no real advantage to using one of these products over another other than flavor. The proper choice for the best oil to be used depends on the patient and the flavor being incorporated. Peanut oil should not be used in patients who may be allergic to peanuts. Sweet almond oil essentially has no flavor of its own, so it is easy to work with. Corn oil is a good choice when preparing an oral liquid for a canine, as dogs enjoy the taste of it and it mixes well with meat flavors without taking away from the flavor being added.

AQUEOUS DILUTING AGENTS

Aqueous diluting agents include aromatic waters and syrups. Aromatic waters are used as diluting agents for water-soluble chemicals and salts. They are not very useful in masking the taste of bad-tasting medications. Peppermint water, purified or distilled water, and preserved water are commonly used aqueous diluents. Syrups are especially useful as diluting agents because they serve as a solvent as well as a sweetening and flavoring vehicle. Some syrups are also a popular choice because of their colloidal properties. Flavored syrups are usually made up of simple syrup and an added flavoring agent. Examples of commonly used syrups include acacia syrup, cherry syrup, raspberry syrup, simple syrup, and Karo® syrup.

HYDROALCOHOLIC DILUTING AGENTS

Hydroalcoholic diluting agents are used when a substance is soluble either in water or in dilute alcohol. The most used form of this type of diluting agent is the elixir, which is made of 25 percent alcohol. Formulas are available for nonmedicated elixirs that can be prepared and then used as a diluting agent, according to the physicochemical properties of the drug being compounded.

ALCOHOLIC DILUTING AGENTS

Alcoholic diluting agents are approximately 50 percent alcohol and are used when a chemical is soluble in a strong alcohol. Tinctures and spirits, when nonmedicated, are the only two types of alcoholic diluting agents used as diluents. Some are available commercially, while others will be made in the pharmacy as needed for compounding medications.

Suspending Agents

A suspending agent is used when a drug is insoluble. The drug's particle size is reduced and then evenly suspended by using the principle of geometric dilution in the suspending vehicle before being brought to final volume with the diluting agent. Common suspending agents include acacia, methylcellulose products, Ora-Plus®, Karo® syrup, and fixed oils. **Micronized** silica gel is one of the most important suspending agents used when compounding oils for oral preparations. The benefits of using silica gel include the facts that it will not discolor the oils and it will allow for easier dispersion of flavors as well as insoluble sweeteners. It is usually used in concentrations of four to six percent. Xanthan gum, a cane sugar derivative, is also an excellent suspending agent due to its natural sweetening and mucilaginous properties. Xanthan gum is usually added in varying concentrations ranging from 0.2 percent to 1 percent. Choice of the proper agent will depend on the physical properties of each of the chemicals and/or excipients contained in the formula.

micronize
to reduce particles to just a few microns in diameter

Determining How Much Flavor

The amount of flavor to be added to any formulation will depend on several factors. Different manufacturers of flavors will produce different concentrations. As a general rule, flavoring agents are added in concentrations ranging from one drop per 1 ml to one drop per 5 ml. Many times, the company that provides the flavoring agent will include a recommendation for the amount of its product to be added. Each individual patient must be considered as well. A newborn patient will not require as much flavoring as a five-year-old. The geriatric patient may require added flavoring due to a possible decline in taste and smell perception. If it is a veterinary compound, the type of animal the prescription is for is important to know as well. Dogs like sweetness and strong aromas, whereas cats will not take a product that is overly sweet or has too strong of an aroma. The drug being incorporated is another factor. If the drug is extremely bitter, then the formulation may require that added sweeteners be used. Likewise, if the drug has little or no taste, very little sweetening is necessary. If the drug possesses a definite odor, additional flavoring may be necessary to mask the smell.

Coloring

Proper coloring of the prescription is equally important. It is not always necessary to color a product, but if a coloring agent is used it should match the flavor of the product. Some patients may have sensitivities or allergies to certain dyes. This should be confirmed beforehand. There are sources of flavoring agents that are dye-free, and these should be considered for the patient who cannot tolerate a certain dye. In any case, the amount of color added to the formulation should be minimal so that the final product is moderately light in color.

In addition to having a list of flavors and their respective pH levels, every pharmacy that offers flavoring should have a compilation of flavors and their recommended uses. These charts are available from various sources, including chemical companies and flavoring manufacturers. There are basically two types of lists. One will provide different types of drugs or drug classes and the most effective choices for flavoring them. The other will provide a list of patient types, both animal and human, and the general preferences of these patients. Referring to this invaluable information source can make a significant difference in producing the best possible preparation of the active ingredient and in benefitting the patient for whom it is prescribed.

Most flavor choices for humans will be made on individual preference with regard to medications being compounded and the appropriate flavors suggested for such products. Since there is such a wide variety of animal patients, the suggested flavors for these patients are based more on species, as indicated in the following chart:

Following are two such (abbreviated) charts (Tables 10-1 and 10-2):

TABLE 10-1 Flavoring Table

Drug Category	Preferred Flavors
Antibiotics	Cherry, pineapple, orange, raspberry, banana, vanilla, butterscotch, strawberry, tutti-frutti, chocolate, marshmallow, bubblegum
Antihistamines	Apricot, cherry, cinnamon, grape, raspberry, root beer, teaberry, lemon, lemon-lime
Barbiturates	Banana-pineapple, cinnamon, peppermint, orange, wintergreen, lime, root beer
Decongestants and Expectorants	Anise, apricot, butterscotch, cherry, strawberry, lemon, maple, orange, raspberry, tutti-frutti, chocolate-marshmallow
Electrolyte Solutions Geriatrics	Cherry, grape, lemon-lime, raspberry, wild cherry syrup, lime, port wine, sherry wine, root beer, strawberry, tutti-frutti, crème de menthe

TABLE 10-2 Veterinary Flavoring Table

Animal	Suggested Flavors
Birds	Tutti-frutti, pina colada, grape, orange, banana, raspberry, molasses (Combinations of fruit flavors work well also.)
Dogs	Bacon, bacon with other meat flavors, beef, liver, chicken, turkey, cheese, peanut butter, *artificial* chocolate, cod liver oil, molasses, raspberry, strawberry, bubblegum
Cats	Fish, fish liver, tuna, cod liver oil, liver, salmon, beef, chicken, cheese, cheese with fish flavors, bacon, butter, butterscotch, marshmallow, molasses
Ferrets	Chocolate, peanut butter, molasses, fish, beef, liver, bacon, chicken, banana, strawberry, watermelon, apple, peas, tutti-frutti
Chinchillas	Banana, tutti-frutti
Horses	Apple, caramel, cherry, molasses, butterscotch, maple, peppermint, sweets
Chickens and Geese	Vanilla, butternut, watermelon, milk, corn, cantaloupe
Rabbits	Carrot, celery, lettuce, banana crème, vanilla butternut, pineapple
Guinea Pigs	Celery, pumpkin, lettuce, carrot, banana crème
Rodents	Lemon, banana crème, cheese, peanut butter, vanilla, butternut
Reptiles	Lemon, banana crème, cheese, peanut butter, vanilla, butternut
Bears	Honey, licorice, chocolate, vanilla
Sea Lions	Medication inserted into a fish

SUMMARY

Successful flavoring of medications is an art form that is improved by experience. It is a valuable service that can be offered to physicians and patients alike. Not only is proper flavoring an important step in making a medication more palatable, it can also mean the difference between a patient being compliant or noncompliant in his prescription therapy.

CHAPTER TERMS

idiosyncrasies
unusual individual reactions to food or a drug

micronize
to reduce particles to just a few microns in diameter

miscible
susceptible to being mixed

palatable
pleasing to the taste

receptors
a molecular structure within a cell or on the surface characterized by selective binding of a specific substance and a specific physiologic effect that accompanies the binding

therapeutic
a desired effect pertaining to the art of healing

CHAPTER 10

CHAPTER REVIEW QUESTIONS

1. What name refers to the famous experiment where a bell was rung for a dog to begin salivating?
   a. Rorschash
   b. Pavlov
   c. Freudian
   d. Clark Rule

2. If "like" base flavorings are not compatible with the base of the compound, what happens to the mixture?
   a. the flavor becomes intense
   b. the flavor will develop a "warmth" to it
   c. degradation
   d. becomes a suspension

3. Sour taste is caused by hydrogen ions and characterized by
   a. acids
   b. tannins
   c. lactones
   d. all of the above

4. The viscosity of highly concentrated sugar solutions may slow down the rate of dissolution of a drug. It is advisable to dissolve the active ingredient in what type of solution first?
   a. aqueous
   b. alcohol
   c. sugar-free suspension
   d. pH balanced

5. A cooling sensation is due to
   a. negative charged ions in the flavoring
   b. positive charged ions in the flavoring
   c. lack of sugar in the flavoring
   d. negative heat of a solution

6. True or false: Coloring a bubblegum-flavored medication pink is an example of recognizing the psychological influence of the senses other than taste.
   a. true
   b. false

7. Trye of false: Monosodium glutonate is an example of a flavor filler.
   a. true
   b. false

8. What are the four basic taste types?

9. Which method uses a stronger flavor to overpower the original flavor?

10. **Critical Thinking** Name and describe the five flavoring techniques.

Resources and References

1. Allen, Loyd V. Jr., Ph.D. *The Art, Science, and Technology of Pharmaceutical Compounding*. Washington, DC: Published by the American Pharmaceutical Association, 1998.
2. *International Journal of Pharmaceutical Compounding*. Houston, TX.
3. *Secundum Artem*. Minneapolis, MN: Paddock Laboratories.

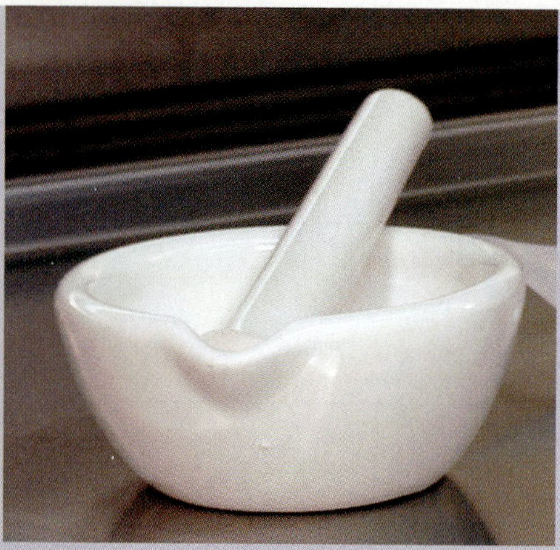

CHAPTER 11

Veterinary Compounding

Learning Objectives

After completing this chapter, you should be able to:

- Identify the aspects of compounding medications for animals.
- List guidelines for establishing a working relationship with veterinarians.
- Outline regulatory issues and precautions that should be met.
- Formulate suggestions for choosing the best route of administration with regard to size and species of the animal to be treated.

INTRODUCTION

The extemporaneous compounding of prescription medication for use in the treatment of animals is an area of pharmacy that offers unique opportunities for the compounding specialist. In this distinct arena of compounding, the pharmacist and technician will perform the true art of compounding medications. Not every compounding setting should or will compound veterinary medications. Those who choose to provide this service should be extensively trained, educated in current clinical information with regard to veterinary medicine, and familiar with veterinary regulatory issues and required business structures.

Working with Veterinarians

Historically, veterinarians have practiced medicine independently of other health care professionals. The dispensing of prescription medications for animals was predominantly done in the veterinarian's office or the animal hospital. This part of veterinary medicine served as a lucrative source of income for the veterinary practice. For this reason, many veterinarians may feel threatened by the services and products offered by a compounding pharmacy. A professional relationship built on trust must be established between the compounding pharmacy staff and the veterinarian if the compounding pharmacy is to succeed in this area. The approach toward the vet should be one that will offer service and solutions to enhance the veterinary practice, and not one that will take business away from the veterinarian, resulting in a reduced profit margin for his practice.

The compounding of veterinary medications for animals should be limited to specialized dosage forms, unique dosages that are not readily available to the vet, combination therapies that will improve treatment and compliancy, and similar situations. A pharmacy specializing in the compounding of veterinary medication should be an extension of the veterinary practice, offering solutions otherwise unobtainable by the veterinarian. A compounding pharmacy should not stock commercially available veterinary products such as heartworm meds, de-worming products, animal vaccines, flea and tick preparations, or commercially available prescription medications for animals.

If a relationship is built on this foundation and nurtured with care, the veterinarian and his staff will come to view the compounding pharmacy as a dependable source for supplying their patients with sought-after treatments and therapies that they would otherwise not have access to. All functions performed with regard to veterinary medicine should be done with the highest standard of quality in order for the veterinarian to place his trust in the pharmacy's compounding ability and eventually come to rely on the services and solutions the pharmacy offers.

Compounding Prescriptions for Veterinary Use

In order for a compounding pharmacy to properly fill veterinary medications, the pharmacists and technicians must become familiar with common terms associated with veterinary medicine and not used in human medicine. For example, the Latin abbreviation **s.i.d.** is used for once-a-day dosing. Since this term is not used in human medicine, it can be misinterpreted, resulting in a medication error. Likewise, it is important that the pharmacy staff develop a basic knowledge of veterinary pharmacology in order to choose the appropriate drug form, vehicle, preservatives, flavoring agents, etc., to properly meet the patient's individual needs.

s.i.d.
a Latin dosing term used in veterinary medicine and indicating that a medication is to be given once a day

The compounding pharmacy that specializes in veterinary compounding of medications should have adequate reference sources for the drugs used in treating animals. These would include Internet sites, as well as books such as *Handbook of Veterinary Drugs* by Dana G. Allen, John K. Pringle, Dale A. Smith, with Kirby Pasloske; and *Veterinary Drug Handbook* by Donald C. Plumb. Other valuable resource books that should be easily accessible are *Trissel's Stability of Compounded Formulations*, *The Merck Veterinary Manual*, and *Remington's Pharmaceutical Sciences*. There are many other journals and books that contain information for prescribing medications in animals. Although it is not necessary to have every book in the pharmacy's library, it is advisable to be familiar with the different sources and the types of information they provide, as well as how to access the knowledge contained within.

Commercially available medications used in the treatment of animals often have names similar to those used for human use. For example, Anapryl is an anti-psychotic agent used to treat dementia in geriatric canines. Although the spelling is different, the name sounds very much like enalapril, a human drug used for the treatment of heart disease (also commonly used in animals). If the staff is familiar with commonly used medications and their intended treatment for animals, they will be aware of such potentials for error. It is not always safe to assume that a human FDA-approved medication is to be used in an animal to treat the same disease state for which it is intended for humans. One example of this is the drug piroxicam, which is generally used for pain and inflammation in humans, but may be used to shrink some forms of cancerous tumors in canines. As with any area of the practice of pharmacy, it is never safe or appropriate to make assumptions about prescription medication.

WORKPLACE WISDOM

Errors that can easily occur with telephoned prescription orders can be avoided by conforming the spelling of the drug being ordered.

Although many drugs used in humans may also be used in animals, there are some major differences in the ways in which the medications are metabolized and distributed in animals. These same medications may be metabolized differently from species to species. For example, there are important differences between cats and dogs, and therefore medication doses should not be indiscriminately extrapolated from one to the other. Proper dosing of medications for each species is listed in the aforementioned books, and these resources should be referenced routinely.

Regulations

Regulatory issues in veterinary medicine are something else to consider before making the decision to compound medications for animals. There are basically two types of compounding for veterinary use. The first category is for those medications which are prepared by using FDA-approved veterinary and human medications and is covered under The Animal Medicinal Drug Use Clarification Act (AMDUCA) of 1994. The second category involves the compounding of prescriptions from bulk chemicals, which is not covered under *AMDUCA*. The FDA views this second type of extemporaneous compounding as illegal and is currently attempting to put an end to it. However, until a law is passed that makes this practice illegal, regulatory discretion must be exercised by the compounding agency following the provisions of the Compliance Policy Guide (*CPG*) for the Compounding of Drugs for Use in Animals. The **CPG** states that the veterinarian is responsible for ensuring that there is a legitimate medical need, identified as follows:

CPG
Compliance Policy Guide—regulatory provision guide for compounding drugs for the use in animals, set forth by the Federal Drug Administration

extra-label use
the use of FDA-approved medication for the treatment of a disease other than that for which it is intended and labeled. Any human drug used in the treatment of animals is considered to be "extra-label." All compounded medications fall under this category as well

- A need exists for an appropriate dosage regimen for the species, age, size, or medical condition of the patient; and
- There is no marketed, approved animal drug that can be used as labeled or in an "**extra-label**" manner of approved human drug; or there is some other rare extenuating circumstance; for example, the approved drug cannot be obtained in time to treat the animal(s) in a timely manner, or there is a medical need for alternate excipients.

After the foregoing determinations are made, the following criteria should be met and precautions observed:

The compounded product may be dispensed by the veterinarian in the course of his practice or by a pharmacist, who must have a prescription from a veterinarian. The CPG encourages veterinarians to "exercise professional judgment to determine when compounding requires the services of a pharmacist." Professional assistance is appropriate when the complexity of compounding exceeds the veterinarian's knowledge, skill, facilities, or available equipment.

The veterinarian should take measures to ensure that no illegal residues occur when a compounded product is used in food-producing animals, that an extended period is assigned for withdrawal from medication, and that steps are taken to ensure that assigned time frames are observed.

A pharmacist compounding for a veterinary patient must adhere to the National Association of Boards of Pharmacy Good Compounding Practices (**GCP**), or to equivalent state good compounding practice regulation, except where provisions conflict with this GCP. Among other practices, pharmacists should keep records of compounding formulas, logs of compounded items and specific ingredients, records of assurance of quality of raw materials, and information on adverse effects and product failures. Pharmacists should label compounded products with expiration dates that do not exceed the prescribed period of treatment, and with withdrawal times furnished by the prescribing veterinarian.

GCP
Good Compounding Practices—state or federal practice regulations for compounding pharmacists

LABELING REQUIREMENTS

The label of a compounded veterinary prescription should contain the following information when filled by a pharmacist:

- Name and address of veterinary practitioner.
- Active ingredient(s).
- Date dispensed and expiration date (not to exceed length of prescribed treatment unless the veterinarian can establish the rationale for a later expiration date).
- Directions for use, including the class and species or identification of the animal(s); and the dose, frequency, route of administration, and duration of therapy.
- Cautionary statements specified by the veterinarian, and/or pharmacist, including all appropriate warnings to ensure safety of humans handling the drugs.
- Veterinarian's specified withdrawal and discard time(s) for meat, milk, eggs, or any food that might be derived from the treated animal(s). (While the veterinarian is responsible for setting the withdrawal time, he may use relevant information provided by a pharmacist in setting the time.)
- Name and address of the dispenser, serial number and date of order or its filling.
- Any other applicable requirements of state or federal law.

Note: It is also necessary to include on all prescriptions for animals the following **Veterinary prescription legend:** "Caution: Federal Law Restricts this Drug to Use by or on the Order of a Licensed Veterinarian."

veterinary prescription legend
"Caution: Federal Law Restricts this Drug to Use by or on the Order of a Licensed Veterinarian." This statement must be included on the label of all manufactured veterinary prescription products

Based on these guidelines and regulations, the choices made for filling prescriptions for animals should be made in the following order:

1. Use of a veterinary, FDA-approved product as it is labeled.
2. Use of a veterinary or human, FDA-approved product in an extra-label manner.
3. Compounding medication using a veterinary or human, FDA-approved product.
4. Compounding medication using bulk, raw chemicals.

Summarizing this information, the decision to compound medicinal agents for animals should be made with extreme caution. Factors in making this determination include the absence of an FDA-approved veterinary product, the identification of an immediate need, and the specific needs of an individual patient (e.g., flavoring; special vehicles; appropriate strengths that are not commercially available; special dosage forms; sensitivities to certain excipients such as proteins, dyes, or preservatives). The FDA's main objective for enforcing laws with regard to medications used in the treatment of animals, especially for **food-producing animals**, is public safety.

food-producing animal
an animal that produces food products for human consumption. Examples included in, but not limited to, this category are cattle, pigs, and poultry

As with the extemporaneous compounding of any prescription product, factors with regard to stability, solubility, ease of administration, dosing, beyond-use dating, storage requirements, proper excipient selection, etc., should be taken into consideration before compounding medications for animals. The same guidelines discussed in previous chapters on the extemporaneous compounding of prescription medication should be adhered to when compounding for veterinary use.

Veterinary Considerations

Because animals come in a wide variety of size and species, each prescription should be considered carefully before a route of administration is recommended to the veterinarian or the owner.

ROUTES OF ADMINISTRATION

Most dogs are usually easily medicated with traditional oral dosage forms such as capsules, tablets, or liquids. Snakes, on the other hand, may require some creativity, such as getting the medication into a mouse and then feeding the mouse to the snake. The route of administration will depend on each individual animal. Cats have the potential for presenting the greatest challenge, as their unique personalities widely differ from feline to feline. Some cats will readily take oral liquids, whereas others simply will not tolerate it. Some cats like to have their ears and head rubbed and thus will allow the application of a transdermal gel, while others despise any kind of contact with their head, affectionate or otherwise. It is imperative that the owner be contacted before deciding on which dosage form the medication should be made into.

Combining multiple medications that are given on the same dosing schedule into one dosage unit will make administration easier and less stressful for both the patient and the owner. This may also ensure better compliancy and prove to be more cost effective for the owner. Of course, this must be approved by the veterinarian first, and the drugs should be researched for compatibility before this suggestion is made.

OWNER CONSIDERATIONS

The owner should also be considered in the dosage form choices. An elderly person with declining eyesight may have trouble reading the dosage lines on an oral or topical syringe. The pet owner who may be physically challenged in some way may also have difficulty dispensing medications from these types of syringes. The handling of very small capsules may also be too much of a challenge for some owners. Cost is sometimes a major consideration for people; therefore, the least expensive way to compound the medication should be evaluated and offered. In addition to considering ease of administration, the owner and other humans or pets in the house should be thought of as well. This is especially true when compounding dangerous or harmful substances such as chemotherapeutic agents for an animal. The owner should be instructed on safe handling methods of the medication and proper disposal of the excrement from the treated animal. Parents should be advised to store all prescription medication out of the reach of children and should use caution when using topical dosage forms where transference can occur if a child handles the pet.

MEDICATION FLAVORING

Each animal has preferred tastes unique to its species. For example, birds tend to like sweet, fruity flavors; dogs and cats generally like meat, fish, or poultry; horses and cattle prefer sweets and grasses; ferrets will eat fish, fruits, and sweet stuff; and gerbils and rabbits prefer fruits and vegetables. That being said, it is not a good idea to make assumptions about a particular species, such as "All cats like tuna." It is important to establish the animal's favorite foods by communicating with the owner before deciding what form and flavor should be prepared.

DOSAGE FORMS

The choices for dosage forms range far beyond the traditional tablet, capsule, or liquid. Transdermal gels, topicals, suppositories, otic and ophthalmic preparations, and chewable treats are among the commonly compounded formulations. As mentioned earlier with the snake example, it may be necessary to use creativity when deciding on the best dosage form. An animal that has a meat protein sensitivity, but whose owner's preferred dosage form is the chewable treat, may require the formulation of a base not made from meat products. Medicated peanut butter troches might be an appropriate alternative. Certain medications may cause a physical reaction from the gelatin contained in the base of the chewable treat (such as from potassium citrate). A liquid could easily be made, but that may not be a good option for either the animal or the owner. An alternative possibility may be, again, the peanut butter troche base, or a base could be prepared using a mixture of hydrogenated vegetable chips and vegetable shortening such as Crisco®. Artificial chocolate products like carob may also be used if appropriate.

Unique Challenges and Suggestions

- An injured bear in the wild that is in need of an antibiotic could be treated by compounding the medication into a sweetened liquid, then pouring the suspension on something like sponge cake and leaving it within close (not too close) proximity of the bear.
- An aggressive animal, such as a lion or tiger at the local zoo, in need of an ophthalmic preparation could have the medication instilled in the affected eye by a squirt gun rather than a standard eye-drop bottle. This method may prove to be safer for the handler and may allow the animal to be treated without the use of tranquilizers.
- Seals, dolphins, whales, and such need only have the proper medication placed inside of a fish just before feeding in order to be successfully treated.
- Domesticated birds may have medications added to their water supply.

SUMMARY

The choices are endless, and a compounding team of pharmacist and technician is encouraged to "think outside of the box" to come up with successful solutions to the problems associated with administering medications to animals.

CHAPTER TERMS

CPG
Compliance Policy Guide—regulatory provision guide for compounding drugs for the use in animals, set forth by the Federal Drug Administration

extra-label use
the use of FDA-approved medication for the treatment of a disease other than that for which it is intended and labeled. Any human drug used in the treatment of animals is considered to be "extra-label" All compounded medications fall under this category as well

food-producing animal
an animal that produces food products for human consumption. Examples included in, but not limited to, this category are cattle, pigs, and poultry

GCP
Good Compounding Practices—state or federal practice regulations for compounding pharmacists

s.i.d.
a Latin dosing term used in veterinary medicine and indicating that a medication is to be given once a day

veterinary prescription legend
"Caution: Federal Law Restricts this Drug to Use by or on the Order of a Licensed Veterinarian." This statement must be included on the label of all manufactured veterinary prescription products

CHAPTER 11

CHAPTER REVIEW QUESTIONS

1. For veterinary prescriptions, s.i.d. means
   a. every other day
   b. once a day
   c. six times per day
   d. four times per day

2. Veterinary compounds from bulk chemicals are regulated by
   a. AMDUCA 94
   b. CSA
   c. FDCA
   d. none of the above

3. According to regulations, the first choice for filling prescriptions for animals should be
   a. use of a veterinary, FDA-approved product as it is labeled
   b. compounding medication using bulk, raw chemicals
   c. use of a veterinary or human, FDA-approved product in an extra-label manner
   d. compounding medication using a veterinary or human, FDA-approved product

4. Generally speaking, which types of animals prefer "sweet" tastes?
   a. dogs and cats
   b. snakes and frogs
   c. cows and ferrets
   d. rabbits and bears

5. Which of the following could be used as a dosage form when compounding veterinary medications for a specific type of animal?
   a. suppository
   b. mouse
   c. otic solution
   d. all of the above

6. True or false: It is appropriate for any pharmacy to compound veterinary medications.
   a. true
   b. false

7. True or false: The purpose of GCP and CPG with regard to veterinary compounding is to provide regulation and guidelines.
   a. true
   b. false

8. What are some of the factors that must be considered before determining the best route of administration for an individual animal?

9. What are four of the unique dosage forms commonly compounded for veterinary use?

10. **Critical Thinking** Why is it necessary to consider the pet owner before compounding a prescription?

Resources and References

1. Compounding of drugs for use in animals. *Compliance Policy Guides Manual*. Division of Compliance Policy/Office of Enforcement, Food and Drug Administration, Washington, D.C., 2004.
2. Bone, Claire, PharmD. A Simplified Guide to Veterinary Compounding. *International Journal of Pharmaceutical Compounding*. Vol. 5 No. 2. Edmond, OK: self-published (IJ PC), 2001.
3. Jordan, Dinah, RPh. Compounding for Animals—A Bird's-Eye View. *International Journal of Pharmaceutical Compounding*. Vol. 1 No. 4, 1997.

APPENDIX A

Answers

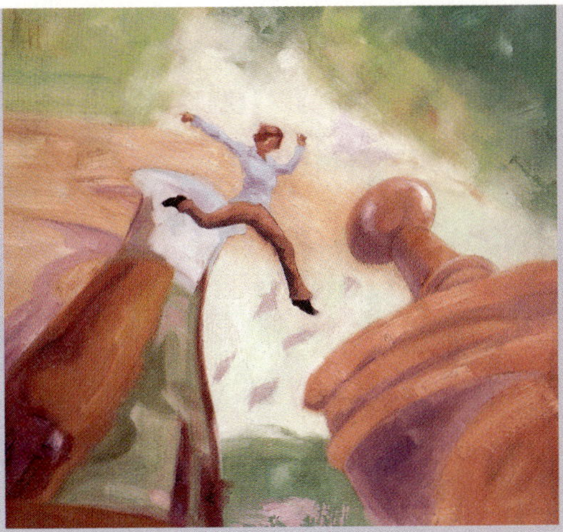

CHAPTER 1
Introduction to Compounding

ANSWERS TO CHAPTER REVIEW QUESTIONS

1. b. pharmacy
2. c. liquid
3. a. radioactive
4. c. avicel
5. d. all of the above
6. a. true
7. a. true
8. beef, chicken, tuna, liver
9. Some drugs have been discontinued; compounding can reduce negative side effects; and others.
10. answers will vary

CHAPTER 2
Compounding Practices and Considerations

ANSWERS TO CHAPTER REVIEW QUESTIONS

1. c. careful, concise
2. c. Always use the numeral 0 before any fraction.
3. a. shelf life
4. d. both b and c
5. b. geometric dilution
6. a. true
7. b. false
8. Remington's, The Merck Manual, US Pharmacopeia, Facts and Comparisons.
9. solubility, stability, shelf life, storage, pH
10. answers will vary

Chapter 3
Facilities, Equipment, and Supplies

ANSWERS TO CHAPTER REVIEW QUESTIONS

1. b. marketing
2. a. every one to seven days
3. d. adaptacaps
4. a. in cabinets with doors, turned upside down
5. c. homogenizer
6. a. true
7. b. false
8. answers will vary
9. Separate from other work flow.
10. answers will vary

Chapter 4
Quality Assurance and Record Keeping

ANSWERS TO CHAPTER REVIEW QUESTIONS

1. c. FDA
2. d. an SOP
3. b. quality control
4. a. USP or NF
5. b. the formulation record
6. a. true
7. b. false
8. To document pharmacy personnel initial and ongoing training and validation.
9. SOPs, recipe sheets, equipment maintenance records
10. answers will vary

Chapter 5
Capsules, Tablets, and Powders

ANSWERS TO CHAPTER REVIEW QUESTIONS

1. b. a capsule
2. a. a tablet
3. c. dosing is set amount
4. d. both b and c
5. c. 60 mg to 100 mg
6. a. true
7. b. false
8. 8
9. placed under the tongue
   dissolve in body fluids
   placed in the cheek pouch to dissolve
10. answers will vary, but may include . . . when a fixed oil is necessary either to dissolve or suspend the drug or because the chemical is stable only in a fixed oil environment and for pharmaceutical elegance also when a drug is light sensitive

Chapter 6
Lozenges, Troches, Sticks, and Suppositories

ANSWERS TO CHAPTER REVIEW QUESTIONS

1. b. chewable
2. a. uniform
3. d. all of the above
4. a. antitussives
5. c. petrolatum
6. b. false
7. a. true
8. molds, hotplate, beaker, thermometer, stirring rods, tongs, grater, spatula, foil wraps, cardboard sleeves
9. lip balm
10. medication can be mistaken as candy. . . .

Chapter 7
Solutions, Suspensions, and Emulsions

ANSWERS TO CHAPTER REVIEW QUESTIONS

1. b. 5
2. c. two phased
3. a. to prevent microbial contamination
4. a. glycerin
5. d. all of the above
6. a. true
7. a. true
8. oral liquid solutions, topical solutions, syrups, elixirs, and aromatic waters
9. the act of reducing a drug to a fine powder
10. drug concentration and solubility, pH of the vehicle and pKa of the drug, taste, and stability. . . .

Chapter 8
Ointments, Creams, Pastes, and Gels

ANSWERS TO CHAPTER REVIEW QUESTIONS

1. b. 25%
2. a. enhance the viscosity of the preparation
3. c. stiffeners
4. c. levigation
5. d. all of the above
6. b. false
7. a. true
8. the oil layer of the micelle is easily absorbed through the outer layer of skin (micelle is a large water drop surrounded by oil formation)
9. the degree of skin penetration and the relationship of water to the base composition.
10. ingredients are placed in a zip lock bag (or similar) and kneaded

Chapter 9
Opthalmic, Otic, and Nasal Preparations

ANSWERS TO CHAPTER REVIEW QUESTIONS

1. b. to help break up the earwax
2. c. in the freezer
3. a. a buffer
4. b. after sterilization
5. a. 4–8
6. a. true
7. a. true
8. because excess or unwanted fluid moves from the inner ear canal into the outer ear canal where it will drain out, thus releasing pressure and discomfort that the patient can experience with ear infections
9. Generic or Chemical Name of the Active Ingredients, Date prepared, Strength and/or Quantity, Pharmacy Lot Number, Beyond Use Dating (Expiration Date), Storage Requirements, Instructions for Use
10. answers can vary

Chapter 10
Medication Flavoring

ANSWERS TO CHAPTER REVIEW QUESTIONS

1. b. Pavlov
2. c. degradation
3. d. all of the above
4. a. aqueous
5. d. negative heat of a solution
6. a. true
7. b. false
8. salt, sweet, bitter, sour
9. Overshadowing
10. Blending, Physical, Chemical, Overshadowing, Physiological . . .

Chapter 11
Veterinary Compounding

ANSWERS TO CHAPTER REVIEW QUESTIONS

1. b. once a day
2. d. none of the above
3. a. use of a veterinary, FDA-approved product as it is labeled
4. c. cows and ferrets
5. d. all of the above
6. b. false
7. a. true
8. ease of use, drug compatibility
9. meat flavored oral liquids, transdermal gels, multi-med capsules, chewable treats
10. cost, handling/reading the compound, storage, animal's preferences

Index

F

G

N

O

P

T

X

Z